Textbook of
Pediatric Advanced Life Support

 American Heart Association

 American Academy of Pediatrics

Editor

Leon Chameides, MD, FAAP
Director, Pediatric Cardiology
Hartford Hospital, and
University of Connecticut
 Health Center
Hartford, Connecticut

Contributing Editors

Ronald S. Bloom, MD, FAAP
Director of Neonatology
Drew Postgraduate
 Medical School
Los Angeles, California

Deborah L. Burkett, EdD
Curriculum Developer
 and Planner
Department of Pediatrics
Harbor UCLA Medical Center
UCLA School of Medicine
Los Angeles, California

Frederick W. Campbell, MD, FAAA
Department of Anesthesia
Children's Hospital of Philadelphia
 and Hospital of the University
 of Pennsylvania
Philadelphia, Pennsylvania

Peter R. Holbrook, MD, FAAP
Director, Critical Care Medicine
Children's Hospital
Washington, District of Columbia

Julius Landwirth, MD, JD, FAAP
Director, Department
 of Pediatrics
Hartford Hospital
Hartford, Connecticut

Robert C. Luten, MD, FAAP
Director, Pediatric
 Emergency Services
University Hospital
Jacksonville, Florida

James H. McCrory, MD
Director, Pediatric Critical Care
University Hospital
Jacksonville, Florida

Richard J. Melker, MD, PhD, FAAP
Director, Division of
 Emergency Medicine
University of Florida
Gainesville, Florida

Richard A. Schieber, MD, FAAP
Director, Pediatric Critical
 Care Medicine
Emory University School
 of Medicine
Atlanta, Georgia

Alan Jay Schwartz, MD, MSEd
Department of Anesthesia
Children's Hospital of Philadelphia
 and Hospital of the University
 of Pennsylvania
Philadelphia, Pennsylvania

James S. Seidel, MD, PhD, FAAP
Chief, Division of
 Ambulatory Pediatrics
Harbor UCLA Medical Center
Los Angeles, California

Ann E. Thompson, MD, FAAP
Director, Pediatric ICU
Children's Hospital
Pittsburgh, Pennsylvania

Robert E. Wood, MD, PhD, FAAP
Director, Pediatric
 Pulmonary Division
University of North Carolina
Chapel Hill, North Carolina

Arno L. Zaritsky, MD, FAAP
Director, Pediatric Critical Care
University of North Carolina
Chapel Hill, North Carolina

Prepared under the direction of the
Subcommittee on Pediatric Resuscitation

Chairman
James S. Seidel, MD, PhD

Members
Robert C. Luten, MD

James H. McCrory, MD

John R. Raye, MD

Arno L. Zaritsky, MD

Of the American Heart Association
Committee on Emergency Cardiac Care

Chairwoman
Judith H. Donegan, MD, PhD

Members
Ramiro Albarran-Sotelo, MD

Allan S. Jaffe, MD

Joseph Ornato, MD

John A. Paraskos, MD

©1988, 1990, American Heart Association

ISBN 0-87493-609-8

Preface

The Pediatric Advanced Life Support Course was developed by a dedicated and hard working committee which it has been my privilege to chair and to whom I am greatly indebted. This textbook is intended as a reference text for the course. Other support materials are provided in the instructor's manual. Each segment has been carefully thought out, written, criticized, and patiently rewritten many times. The course has been tested twice: in Hartford, Connecticut, in December 1985 and in Washington, D.C., in April 1986. Despite this, there are doubtless errors of fact and omission which I leave to others to criticize, research, prove, and correct.

Leon Chameides, MD

Table of Contents

Chapter 8
Immediate Postarrest Stabilization

Chapter 9
Ethical and Legal Aspects
of Cardiopulmonary
Resuscitation in Children

Appendices

He who has saved one life, has saved the whole world.

— *Mishnah Sanhedrin 4:5*

Introduction

And it came to pass, after these things, that the son of the woman, the mistress of the house, fell sick; and his sickness was so sore, that there was no breath left in him. . .and [Elijah] said unto her "Give me thy son." And he took him out of her bosom, and carried him up into the upper chamber where he abode, and laid him upon his own bed. And he cried unto the Lord, and said: "O Lord my God, hast thou also brought evil upon the widow with whom I sojourn, by slaying her son?" And he stretched himself upon the child three times, and cried unto the Lord and said: "O Lord my God, I pray thee, let this child's soul come back into him." And the Lord hearkened unto the voice of Elijah; and the soul of the child came back into him, and he revived.

— *I Kings 17:17–22*
King James Version

Some of the modern concepts of cardiopulmonary resuscitation (CPR) are already evident in this first case report of a pediatric resuscitation. There is a victim (the child) and a bystander (the mother) who makes a correct assessment of the problem and transports the victim to an advanced life support facility (Elijah). The rescuer lies down on the victim (mouth-to-mouth ventilation?), and the victim recovers.

Reanimation, however, remained only a dream for many centuries until Kouwenhoven and associates[1] demonstrated that closed-chest cardiac compressions, in an arrested cardiovascular state, can allow sufficient blood circulation to maintain life until definitive treatment can be provided.

I. Historical Setting

In 1966 The National Academy of Sciences-National Research Council (NAS-NRC) Conference on Cardiopulmonary Resuscitation recommended the training of medical allied health and professional personnel in the techniques of CPR according to the standards of the American Heart Association (AHA).[2] In 1973, at a national conference co-sponsored by the AHA and the NAS-NRC, it was recommended that training in Basic Life Support (BLS), which includes CPR without adjuncts, be extended to the general public.[3] An adult Advanced Cardiac Life Support (ACLS) course was first presented by the American Medical Association in 1974 and was adopted by the American Heart Association in 1975.

No pediatricians were involved in the 1966 or the 1973 National Conferences, and the only reference to infants and children in the resulting standards was a drug dosage chart. In order to correct this omission, the Working Group on Pediatric Resuscitation was formed in 1978 under the auspices of the AHA Subcommittee on Emergency Cardiac Care. This group developed standards in pediatric basic life support (BLS) and guidelines for neonatal resuscitation that were accepted by the 1979 National Conference.[4] The 1985 National Conference boasted three speakers on various aspects of pediatric resuscitation, and three panels (Pediatric BLS, Pediatric Advanced Life Support (ALS), and Neonatal Resuscitation) were presented. These resulted in revised standards for pediatric BLS, revised guidelines in neonatal resuscitation, and the development of pediatric ALS guidelines,[5] all of which were endorsed by the American Academy of Pediatrics.

In December 1983, a National Conference on Pediatric Resuscitation was convened under the auspices of the AHA. In addition to experts in the field, the following organizations were represented: the Section of Pediatric Emergency Medicine and the Committee on the Fetus and Newborn of the American Academy of Pediatrics; the American Academy of Family Physicians; the American College of Cardiology; the American College of Surgeons; the American Medical Association; the American Society of Anesthesiology; the Canadian Heart Foundation; the National Perinatal Association; and the Nurses Association of the American College of Obstetricians and Gynecologists. The conference defined the general content of courses in neonatal and pediatric ALS and stated that 1) courses on pediatric and neonatal ALS were urgently needed and 2) developing standards and administering courses should be under the auspices of the American Heart Association.

II. Why a Separate Course of Pediatric Advanced Life Support?

The major differences between CPR for adults and children are 1) etiologies and mechanisms of the cardiopulmonary arrest and 2), often, the health professionals providing care.

The most common cause of cardiac arrest in adults is a primary cardiac event, and accordingly, a significant portion of the adult ACLS course is devoted to recognizing and treating rhythm disturbances. The causes of cardiac arrest in children are diverse but the final common pathway is usually profound hypoxemia and acidosis, often of respiratory or circulatory origin. Emphasis in the

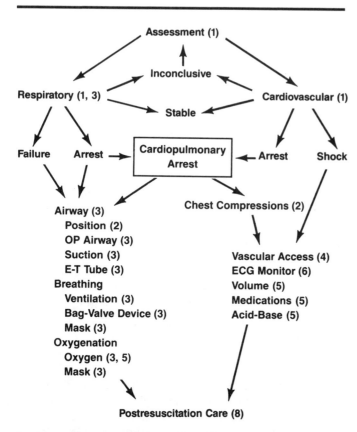

Assessment (1)

Inconclusive

Respiratory (1, 3)   Cardiovascular (1)

Stable

Failure   Arrest → Cardiopulmonary ← Arrest   Shock
                         Arrest

Airway (3)   Chest Compressions (2)
  Position (2)
  OP Airway (3)
  Suction (3)
  E-T Tube (3)   Vascular Access (4)
Breathing   ECG Monitor (6)
  Ventilation (3)   Volume (5)
  Bag-Valve Device (3)   Medications (5)
  Mask (3)   Acid-Base (5)
Oxygenation
  Oxygen (3, 5)
  Mask (3)

Postresuscitation Care (8)

The Resuscitation Process. The numbers in parentheses refer to the chapters in which the information is located.

pediatric course is therefore placed on pre-arrest assessment, anticipatory intervention, and ventilation techniques.

The American Heart Association, through its ACLS courses, has had an enormous impact on the standards, skills, and procedures in the resuscitation of adult victims. These skills and procedures have also raised many questions, and researchers have been stimulated to search for a better understanding of the mechanisms of, and improved techniques in, rescue efforts. Unfortunately, this has not been true of child victims. Health professionals dealing primarily with children have not been reached by the AHA courses since they lack relevance to the pediatric age group. Procedures become systematized through drills provided by formal courses, and their lack has led to the absence of a systematic approach in the resuscitation of infants and children. Compounding this deficiency, equipment and training for the prehospital resuscitation of children is often woefully inadequate despite the fact that a significant portion of emergency calls involve the pediatric age group.[6,7]

III. Overview

This textbook is a companion to the Pediatric Advanced Life Support course, which includes lectures, skill stations, and interactive sessions (see "Appendix C: Overview of the Pediatric Advanced Life Support Course"). The goal of the textbook is to provide the student with an up-to-date reference on various aspects of advanced life support for infants and children, while the goal of the course is to integrate knowledge and motor skills into a clinically useful discipline.

The structure of the text makes the contents of the chapters appear isolated from each other although they, like resuscitation itself, should be viewed as a continuum in *time*:

**Preresuscitation →
Resuscitation → Postresuscitation**

and in *activity*:

Assessment → Action → Reassessment

The resuscitative process involves information presented in many chapters. The relation of text to steps of the resuscitation process is visually displayed at left, beginning with the assessment of the cardiovascular and respiratory systems.

The conclusion of the assessment may be:

1. that the systems are stable, in which case no further action is necessary;
2. that the systems are unstable, in which case action depends on the degree of instability; or
3. that the assessment is inconclusive, in which case the child needs careful observation and repeated assessments.

References

1. Kouwenhoven WB, Jude JR, Knickerbocker GG: Closed chest cardiac massage. *JAMA* 173:1064, 1960.
2. Cardiopulmonary Resuscitation: Statement of the Ad Hoc Committee on Cardiopulmonary Resuscitation of the Division of Medical Sciences-National Research Council. *JAMA* 198:372, 1966.
3. Standards for Cardiopulmonary Resuscitation (CPR) and Emergency Cardiac Care (ECC). *JAMA* 227:833, 1974.
4. Standards and Guidelines for Cardiopulmonary Resuscitation (CPR) and Emergency Cardiac Care (ECC). *JAMA* 244:453, 1980.
5. Standards and Guidelines for Cardiopulmonary Resuscitation (CPR) and Emergency Cardiac Care (ECC). *JAMA* 255:2954, 1986.
6. Seidel JS, Hornbein M, Yuoshiyama K, et al: Emergency medical services and the pediatric patient: Are needs being met? *Pediatrics* 73:769, 1984.
7. Seidel JS: Emergency medical services and the pediatric patient: Are the needs being met? II. Training and equipping emergency medical services providers for pediatric emergencies. *Pediatrics* 78:808,1986.

Recognition of Respiratory Failure and Shock: Anticipating Cardiopulmonary Arrest

Cardiopulmonary arrest in infants and children is not usually a sudden event. Instead, it is often the end-result of a progressive deterioration in respiratory and circulatory function, the final common pathway of which is cardiopulmonary failure, regardless of the underlying disease (Figure 1.1). An arrest can often be prevented if the clinician recognizes symptoms of respiratory failure and/or shock and promptly initiates therapy. This chapter presents guidelines for anticipating cardiopulmonary arrest in infants and children and for establishing priorities in care.

Respiratory failure is a clinical state characterized by inadequate elimination of carbon dioxide and/or inadequate oxygenation of the blood. This may occur because of intrinsic lung or airway disease or because of inadequate respiratory effort (e.g., the patient with apnea or shallow respirations from intracranial pathology). *Shock* is a clinical state characterized by inadequate delivery of oxygen and metabolic substrates to meet the metabolic demands of tissues; note that this definition fails to mention blood pressure. Shock may occur with a normal, increased, or most frequently, decreased cardiac output. Shock may be further classified into compensated and decompensated conditions. In compensated shock, blood pressure is normal. Decompensated shock is characterized by hypotension and, often, by a low cardiac output.

As with shock, respiratory failure is often preceded by a "compensated" state in which the patient is able to maintain adequate gas exchange at the expense of an increase in the work of breathing. This compensated state is characterized by respiratory distress, the use of accessory muscles of respiration, inspiratory retractions, tachypnea, and tachycardia.

Although respiratory failure and shock may begin as clinically distinct syndromes, they progress to an indistinguishable state of cardiopulmonary failure in the final moments before arrest. Their common clinical features are caused by insufficient oxygen delivery to tissues and reduced clearance of metabolites. In shock associated with a low cardiac output state, blood, even though it may be well oxygenated, is delivered too slowly to meet tissue metabolic demand. In advanced respiratory failure, poorly oxygenated blood may be delivered at a normal or elevated flow rate to the tissues. In both cases tissue hypoxia is present. In shock, tissue metabolic demand exceeds oxygen delivery and lactic acid is produced; in respiratory failure, blood carbon dioxide tension increases because pulmonary gas exchange is impaired. Both cases result in acidemia (low blood pH) and tissue acidosis.

Clinical signs of shock and respiratory failure result from end-organ dysfunction caused by tissue hypoxia and acidosis. These include altered levels of consciousness, hypotonia, tachycardia, and weak central (proximal) pulses with absent peripheral pulses. Bradycardia, hypotension, and irregular respirations are late, ominous signs. Cardiopulmonary failure should be suspected in any infant or child who has respiratory distress, severe multiple or blunt trauma, a reduced level of consciousness, cyanosis, or pallor (Table 1.1).

I. Evaluation of Respiratory Performance

Normal ventilation is accomplished with minimal work. The normal respiratory rate decreases with age; it is less

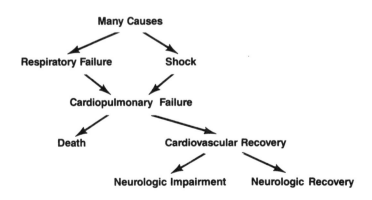

Figure 1.1. Path of various disease states leading to cardiopulmonary failure in infants and children.

Table 1.1. Selected Conditions Requiring a Rapid Cardiopulmonary Assessment

Any of the following:	
____ Respiratory rate	> 60
____ Heart rate	>180 or <80 (under 5 years)
	>160 (over 5 years)
____ Respiratory distress	
____ Trauma	
____ Burns	
____ Cyanosis	
____ Failure to recognize parents	
____ Diminished level of consciousness	
____ Seizures	
____ Fever with petechiae	
____ Admission to an ICU	

than 40 breaths/min in the newborn, approximately 24 breaths/min in the 1-year-old child, and approximately 18 breaths/min in the 18 year old. These rates may vary with excitement, anxiety, or fever. Tidal volume (the volume of each breath) per kg of body weight, however, remains fairly constant throughout life. Tidal volume is assessed clinically by auscultation over the lungs, noting the quality of air movement and the adequacy of chest wall excursion.

Abnormal respirations are classified as too fast (tachypnea), too slow (bradypnea), absent (apnea), and/or associated with an increased work of breathing. Minute ventilation, the product of tidal volume and respiratory rate, may be low (hypoventilation) because each breath is shallow or because too few breaths are taken each minute. Acute respiratory failure results from any pulmonary or neuromuscular disease that impairs the elimination of carbon dioxide (ventilation) and/or oxygen exchange (oxygenation) at the alveolar–capillary membrane.[1] The resultant hypercapnia and/or hypoxemia reflects the severity of respiratory failure.

Possible respiratory arrest should be anticipated in infants and children who have 1) an increased respiratory rate, an increased respiratory effort, or diminished breath sounds, 2) a diminished level of consciousness or response to pain, 3) poor skeletal muscle tone, or 4) cyanosis.

The assessment of respiratory function is based on careful evaluation of respiratory rate, respiratory mechanics, and skin and mucous membrane color as outlined below.

A. Respiratory Rate

Tachypnea may be the first manifestation of respiratory distress in infants. Tachypnea without respiratory distress ("quiet tachypnea") commonly results from nonpulmonary diseases, especially metabolic acidosis associated with shock, diabetic ketoacidosis, inborn errors of metabolism, salicylism, severe diarrhea, and chronic renal insufficiency. Thus, quiet tachypnea is often an attempt to maintain a normal pH by increasing minute ventilation and thereby cause a compensatory respiratory alkalosis.

A slow respiratory rate in an *acutely ill* infant or child is an ominous sign. Causes include hypothermia, fatigue, and central nervous system depression. Fatigue needs to be especially emphasized. An infant breathing at a rate of 80 breaths/min will likely tire; a decreasing respiratory rate is not necessarily a sign of improvement!

B. Respiratory Mechanics

Increased work of breathing is evidenced by nasal flaring and intercostal, subcostal, and suprasternal inspiratory retractions; it may be seen in children with respiratory problems, including airway obstruction and alveolar diseases. As work of breathing increases, a greater proportion of the cardiac output must be delivered to the

respiratory muscles, which in turn produce more carbon dioxide. Respiratory acidosis is followed by metabolic acidosis when the work of breathing exceeds the ability to provide adequate tissue oxygenation.

Head bobbing, stridor, prolonged expiration, and grunting are important signs of altered respiratory mechanics. A bobbing of the head with each breath is often an indication of impending respiratory failure. Extreme inspiratory efforts draw the chest in while thrusting the abdomen out, causing "see–saw" or rocky respirations.

Stridor (an inspiratory, high-pitched sound) is a sign of upper airway obstruction occurring between the supraglottic space and the lower trachea. Causes of upper airway obstruction include 1) congenital abnormalities (e.g., vocal cord paralysis, airway tumor, or cyst), 2) infections (e.g., epiglottitis or croup), and 3) aspiration of a foreign body.

Prolonged expiration, usually accompanied by wheezing, is a sign of bronchial and bronchiolar obstruction and is often caused by bronchiolitis or asthma.

Grunting is produced by premature glottic closure accompanying active chest wall contraction during early expiration. Infants and children grunt to increase airway pressure, thereby preserving or increasing functional residual capacity in diseases that cause accumulation of interstitial or alveolar fluid. Grunting is heard in patients whose disease causes alveolar collapse and loss of lung volume, including patients with pulmonary edema, pneumonia, atelectasis, and adult respiratory distress syndrome.

C. Cyanosis

Cyanosis is a fairly late and inconsistent sign of respiratory failure and is best seen in the mucous membranes of the mouth and nail beds; cyanosis of the extremities alone (peripheral cyanosis) is more likely due to circulatory failure (shock) than to pulmonary failure. Arterial blood gases should be measured whenever a question of serious respiratory impairment exists, even in the absence of cyanosis.

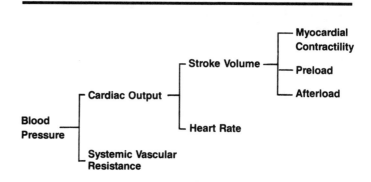

Figure 1.2. Hemodynamic relationships.

II. Evaluation of Cardiovascular Performance

Shock is the failure of the cardiovascular system to adequately perfuse vital organs.[2-4] Failure to deliver critical substrates and remove metabolites leads to anaerobic metabolism, accumulation of acid, and irreversible cellular damage. Death due to cardiovascular collapse may follow shortly; death due to multiple organ system failure resulting from cellular damage may be delayed.

Cardiac output is the volume of blood pumped by the heart each minute (heart rate × stroke volume), while stroke volume is the volume pumped with each beat. Blood pressure is the product of cardiac output and peripheral resistance (Figure 1.2). Organ perfusion is determined by cardiac output and perfusion pressure. Of the variables in Figure 1.2, heart rate and blood pressure can be measured easily; stroke volume and peripheral vascular resistance must be qualitatively assessed by examining pulses and evaluating tissue perfusion.

Although shock is often associated with a low cardiac output, septic and anaphylactic shock may be characterized by an increase in cardiac output and a normal blood pressure.[5] When cardiac output is increased, vascular resistance is low and the patient may appear well perfused, with bounding pulses and a wide pulse pressure. Despite appearing well-perfused, the patient's metabolic demand exceeds the increased oxygen supply, and there is often a mismatch between tissue blood flow and metabolic demand ("distributive shock"). This form of shock may be quite subtle, and a high index of suspicion is required for its recognition. Attention to the assessment signs discussed below and analysis of arterial blood gases should lead to the correct diagnosis.

A. Heart Rate

Normal heart rates in infants and children are given in Chapter 6. Sinus tachycardia (see Chapter 6) is a common response to many types of stress (e.g., anxiety, fever, hypoxia, hypercapnia, or hypovolemia). The presence of tachycardia therefore mandates further evaluation to determine the underlying cause. *Newborns* increase their cardiac output principally by increasing heart rate and, to a lesser extent, by increasing contractility and altering preload and afterload. The primary response of the neonatal heart to hypoxemia often is bradycardia; in older children, tachycardia is the first response. When tachycardia fails to compensate adequately, tissue hypoxia and hypercapnia with acidosis develop and bradycardia ensues. Bradycardia in a distressed child is an ominous sign of impending cardiac arrest.

B. Blood Pressure

As noted previously, blood pressure is determined by cardiac output and peripheral vascular resistance. Normal blood pressure can be maintained as long as the circula-

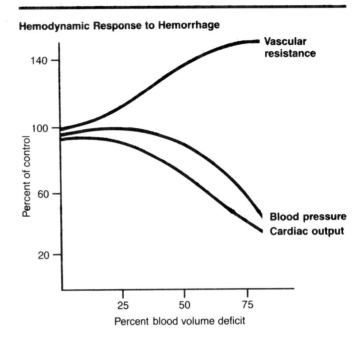

Hemodynamic Response to Hemorrhage

Figure 1.3. Model for cardiovascular response to hypovolemia from hemorrhage.

tion compensates adequately with vasoconstriction, tachycardia, and increased cardiac contractility. When compensation fails, hypotension occurs. Tachycardia persists until cardiac reserve is depleted. Figure 1.3 shows a model for the cardiovascular response to hemorrhagic shock. Although cardiac output falls in an almost linear fashion as blood volume is depleted, blood pressure remains initially unchanged because of increased vascular resistance. Hypotension is a *late and often sudden sign* of cardiovascular decompensation. Even mild hypotension must be taken seriously and treated quickly and vigorously since cardiopulmonary arrest is often close at hand.

Normal blood pressure values for age are given in Figure 1.4. A formula that has been used to approximate a typical systolic blood pressure in children over the age of 2 years is 90 + (2 × age in years). The *lower limit* of systolic blood pressure has been approximated by the formula 70 + (2 × age in years). An observed fall of 10 mmHg in systolic pressure should prompt careful serial evaluations for other signs of shock.

C. Peripheral Circulation

Since sinus tachycardia is a nonspecific sign of shock and hypotension is a late sign, the diagnosis of early shock depends on the clinical assessment of stroke volume and peripheral vascular resistance. This is best accomplished by evaluating the presence and volume of peripheral pulses and the adequacy of end-organ perfusion.

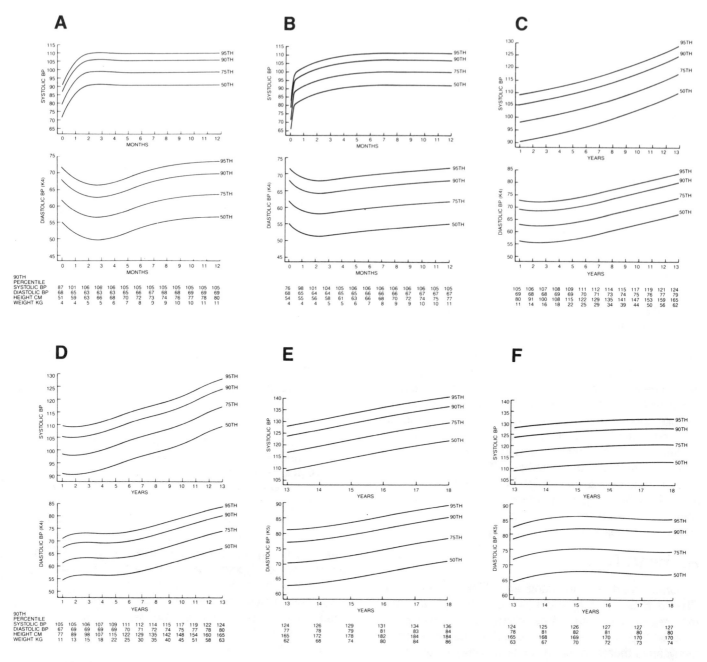

Figure 1.4. Normal blood pressures in infants and children. Age-specific percentiles of blood pressure measurements in A) boys from birth to 12 months, B) girls from birth to 12 months, C) boys from 1 to 13 years, D) girls from 1 to 13 years, E) boys from 13 to 18 years, F) girls from 13 to 18 years. Korotkoff Phase IV used for diastolic blood pressures in A–D; Phase V, in E and F. (From Report of the Second Task Force on Blood Pressure — 1987. *Pediatrics* 79:1, 1987. Reproduced by permission of *Pediatrics*.)

The carotid, axillary, brachial, radial, femoral, dorsalis pedis, and posterior tibial pulses are readily palpable in healthy infants and children. A discrepancy in volume between central and peripheral pulses may be due to vasoconstriction associated with hypothermia, or it may be an early sign of a diminished stroke volume. Pulse volume is related to pulse pressure (difference between systolic and diastolic pressures). As shock progresses, pulse pressure narrows, making the pulse "thready" and, finally, impalpable. Loss of central pulses is a premorbid sign. Early septic shock is a high output state and, in contrast to low-output shock, is often characterized by a wide pulse pressure and, therefore, bounding pulses.

D. End-Organ Perfusion

1. The Skin

End-organ perfusion is evaluated best in the skin, brain, and kidneys. Decreased perfusion of the skin is an *early* sign of shock. Normally, the hands and feet are warm, dry, and pink to the distal phalanx. As cardiac output decreases, the line of demarcation between warmth and coolness ascends toward the trunk.[6] Slow capillary refilling (> 2 seconds) after blanching is evidence of low cardiac output or hypothermia. In testing for capillary refill, the extremity should be lifted slightly above the level of the heart.

Mottling, pallor, poor capillary refill, and peripheral cyanosis indicate poor skin perfusion; acrocyanosis may be normal in the newborn. Severe vasoconstriction causes a grey or ashen color in newborns and pallor in older age groups. The pattern of mottling changes with time and represents variable cutaneous perfusion.

2. The Brain

The signs of brain hypoperfusion exhibited depends on its severity and duration.[7] In children with sudden onset of brain ischemia, few signs of neurologic compromise precede loss of consciousness. Muscular tone is lost, and generalized convulsions and pupillary dilation may occur.

In subacute hypoperfusion, such as shock, symptoms are more insidious. Alteration of consciousness occurs, with confusion and lethargy. An alternating picture of agitation and lethargy is often seen, with the child quiet when undisturbed and combative when procedures are attempted. Infants may be irritable and have a fretful look, weak cry, and wrinkled brow. After 2 months of age, an infant should normally focus on his or her parents' faces. Failure to recognize parents may be an early, ominous sign of cortical hypoperfusion or cerebral dysfunction. This may be obvious only to the parents, who may not be able to describe it any better than to say, "There's something wrong."

More profound degrees of hypoperfusion produce greater changes in the level of consciousness. In decreasing order of levels of consciousness, the child may be:

1. awake,
2. responsive to voice,
3. responsive to pain,
4. unresponsive.

Deep tendon reflexes may be depressed, pupils may be small but reactive, and a crescendo–decrescendo breathing pattern (Cheyne–Stokes) may be apparent.

Hypotonia and intermittent flexor or extensor posturing may occur with prolonged cerebral hypoperfusion or extreme hypoxemia (arterial pO_2 < 30 mmHg).

3. The Kidneys

Urinary output is directly proportional to glomerular filtration rate and renal blood flow. The rate of urinary flow is a good indicator of therapeutic progress, but it is not very helpful in the initial evaluation since the history of urine production in the recent past is often vague and imprecise. Normal urine output is 1–2 mL/kg/hr; a urine flow of < 1 mL/kg/hr in the absence of renal disease, is a sign of poor perfusion. An indwelling urinary catheter facilitates accurate urine flow determination.

III. Rapid Cardiopulmonary Assessment

Recognition of the physiologically unstable infant or child is a critical clinical challenge that can be made by physical examination alone. Laboratory tests are useful adjuncts in evaluating the severity but are not essential in making the diagnosis. Every clinician working with sick children should be able to diagnose pulmonary and circulatory failure and impending cardiopulmonary arrest based on a *rapid cardiopulmonary assessment* (Table 1.2). The rapid cardiopulmonary assessment is a survey whose main goal is to answer the question, "Does this child have pulmonary or circulatory failure that may lead to arrest?" It takes less than half a minute to complete and, by integrating important physical findings, is designed to evaluate pulmonary and cardiovascular integrity through effects on target organs.

Table 1.2. Rapid Cardiopulmonary Assessment

Respiratory Assessment	Cardiovascular Assessment
A. AIRWAY PATENCY	C. CIRCULATION
B. BREATHING	Heart Rate
Rate	Blood Pressure
Air Entry	Peripheral Pulses
Chest rise	Present/absent
Breath sounds	Volume
Stridor	
Wheezing	Skin Perfusion
	Capillary refill time
Mechanics	Temperature
Retractions	Color
Grunting	Mottling
Accessory muscle use	
Nasal flaring	CNS Perfusion
	Recognition of parents
Color	Reaction to pain
	Muscle tone
	Pupil size

The assessment uses the A–B–C approach of cardio-pulmonary resuscitation (the ''ABC's of CPR'').

A. **A**irway: The airway is determined to be either 1) *patent*, 2) *maintainable* with head positioning, suctioning, or adjuncts, or 3) *unmaintainable* and requiring interventions such as removal of a foreign body, intubation, or cricothyrotomy.

B. **B**reathing: Evaluation of breathing focuses on the presence of inspiratory breath sounds, an evaluation of the work of breathing, the adequacy of the tidal volume and resultant chest expansion, and the adequacy of minute ventilation to sustain heart rate and circulation.

C. **C**irculation: An examination of the peripheral circulation qualitatively reveals, the adequacy of cardiac output. The presence and quality of peripheral pulses, capillary refill time, and end-organ perfusion are assessed using criteria discussed previously.

Examination of the ill infant or child does not end when the rapid cardiopulmonary assessment is completed. These patients are often in a dynamic state, and *repeated* assessments are necessary. Repeat evaluations determine whether the patient's clinical condition has deteriorated or is improving in response to therapy.

IV. Priorities in Management

On the basis of the Rapid Cardiopulmonary Assessment, the child is categorized as 1) stable, 2) in questionable respiratory failure or shock, 3) in definite respiratory failure or shock, or 4) in cardiopulmonary failure.

When pulmonary or circulatory failure is suspected but not definitely present, sequential assessments should be performed. Supplemental laboratory studies, especially arterial blood gas analysis and chest x-ray, may be useful. When poor ventilation, oxygenation, or perfusion threatens cardiopulmonary stability, supportive interventions and assessments should be performed promptly and continued until stability is established before attempting a definitive diagnosis.

The child with respiratory distress or well-compensated shock should be approached in a prompt and efficient, yet thoughtful and gentle, manner that minimizes stress and oxygen demand. Supplemental oxygen should be given in a nonthreatening manner whenever possible; several methods may need to be tried. In patients with upper airway obstruction, the child's position of maximal comfort should be respected in order to minimize the work of breathing and optimize airway patency. Normal body temperature should be maintained, and feeding should be withheld.

In patients with respiratory failure, the airway should be secured and adequate ventilation assured with maximum supplemental oxygen (see Chapter 3). In shock, vascular access should be established rapidly (see Chapter 4) and volume expansion and medications given, as necessary (see Chapter 5).

In cardiopulmonary failure, initial priority is given to ventilation and oxygenation. If circulation and perfusion fail to improve rapidly, therapy for shock is given (see Chapter 5).

V. Special Conditions Predisposing to Cardiopulmonary Arrest

Certain conditions that may place infants and children at risk of cardiopulmonary failure deserve special attention. More comprehensive discussions of the pathophysiology and management of these conditions can be found in texts relating to pediatric trauma, emergency, and critical care medicine.

A. Positive-Pressure Ventilation

Cardiovascular collapse due to hypoxemia may occur despite tracheal intubation and positive-pressure ventilation if 1) the endotracheal tube is obstructed, 2) the tube is displaced into the esophagus or main-stem bronchus, 3) a tension pneumothorax is present, or 4) the mechanical ventilation device fails. See Chapter 3 for recognition and management of these problems.

B. Epiglottitis

Acute epiglottitis usually presents before 5 years of age with an acute onset of fever, sore throat, drooling, muffled voice, and inspiratory stridor. The child prefers to lean forward while sitting and holds his or her head in a sniffing position. This preference should be respected and supported; supplemental oxygen can be administered while the child is sitting in the parent's lap. Respiratory arrest can occur from total airway obstruction or a combination of partial airway obstruction and fatigue. If epiglottitis is strongly suspected, the patient should proceed *directly* to the operating room. Such patients deserve definitive airway management by the physician most skillful in managing the difficult airway, since the inflamed, swollen surpraglottis makes intubation difficult. If respiratory arrest occurs, bag-mask ventilation with 100% oxygen should precede any attempt to intubate the patient or to perform emergency tracheotomy or needle cricothyrotomy.

C. Tracheostomy

An infant with a tracheostomy is at high risk for respiratory arrest if a mucous plug obstructs the artificial airway (see Chapter 3). The infant's small tracheal diameter and inability to cry for help compound the possibility of obstruction. Tracheal obstruction should be considered the cause of an arrest in a tracheostomy patient until proven otherwise. If a brief suctioning attempt fails to relieve the obstruction, the tracheostomy tube should be removed immediately. The infant often has enough reserve to breathe spontaneously before the stoma is suctioned and a new tube is inserted. Otherwise, the stoma can be manually occluded and the infant ventilated with a bag and mask prior to orotracheal intubation.

D. Burns

Children with major burns require careful and frequent assessments for shock and respiratory failure. Patients with severe burns of the head and neck may need prompt endotracheal intubation, in order to protect the airway, before edema distorts the anatomy. Carbon monoxide poisoning should be suspected and treated with maximal supplemental oxygen.

E. Trauma

Respiratory failure in children with trauma may occur as a result of central nervous system depression, upper airway obstruction, pneumothorax, pulmonary contusion, or flail chest. Suspected cervical fractures should be treated by neck immobilization until that diagnosis has been excluded. Hemorrhagic shock is most often due to hepatic or splenic injury, but hemothorax, a fractured femur with vascular laceration, scalp lacerations, and intracranial hemorrhage (in the newborn or infant) may be other sites of major blood loss.[8,9]

F. Gastroenteritis

Hypovolemia due to fluid loss secondary to a gastrointestinal infection may cause shock in infants and children. Signs of dehydration precede those of shock and include lethargy, an absence of tearing, dry mucous membranes, and a dry, sometimes doughy, consistency of the skin. Rapid volume expansion is indicated to prevent cardiovascular collapse.

G. Seizures

Seizures may cause respiratory depression, or upper airway obstruction by secretions or prolapse of soft tissues into the hypopharynx. Apnea may result from some medications used to treat the seizures.

H. Critically Ill Patients

All infants and children who require intensive care, including those in an intensive care unit, in an operating room, in an emergency room, or who are in transit within or between hospitals, are at high risk for cardiopulmonary arrest.[10] Cardiopulmonary arrest may result from:

1. the natural history of a life-threatening disease;
2. a complication of therapy;
3. premature withdrawal of support, including mechanical ventilation, supplemental oxygen, or vasoactive drugs; or
4. the accidental withdrawal of such support.

In patients who have recently been resuscitated, cardiovascular instability and arrest may recur because:

1. catecholamines administered during resuscitation have been metabolized and not replaced by a continuous infusion;
2. the inciting event recurs; or
3. hypoxic–ischemic myocardial, pulmonary, or cerebral damage has occurred.

I. Coma

In a comatose infant or child, intubation is required to treat hypoventilation and to provide airway protection. Intracranial hypertension, which may be present in some comatose patients, may be aggravated by intubation by an inexperienced operator. In such situations bag–valve ventilation should be used and tracheal intubation should be postponed until it can be safely performed using muscle relaxants and an anesthetic regimen for neuroinduction. Posturing after head trauma must be considered a sign of increased intracranial pressure. Cushing's triad (bradycardia, hypertension, and apnea) is a very late manifestation, and its absence in children does not exclude the presence of increased intracranial pressure.

References

1. Downes JJ, Fulgencio T, Raphaely RC: Acute respiratory failure in infants and children. *Pediatr Clin North Am* 19:423, 1972.
2. Crone RK: Acute circulatory failure in children. *Pediatr Clin North Am* 27:525, 1980.
3. Perkin RM, Levin DL: Shock in the pediatric patient, Part I. *J Pediatr* 101:163, 1982.
4. Perkin RM, Levin DL: Shock in the pediatric patient, Part II. *J Pediatr* 101:319, 1982.
5. Ellner JJ: Septic shock. *Pediatr Clin North Am* 30:365, 1983.
6. Joly HR, Weil MH: Temperature of the great toe as an indication of the severity of shock. *Circulation* 39:131, 1969.
7. Plum F, Posner JB: *The Diagnosis of Stupor and Coma*, 3 ed. Philadelphia, F.A. Davis Co., 1982.
8. Committee on Trauma: *Advanced Trauma Life Support*. American College of Surgeons, 1981.
9. Eichelberger MR, Randolph JG: Pediatric trauma: An algorithm for diagnosis and therapy. *J Trauma* 23:91, 1983.
10. Von Seggern K, Egar M, Fuhrman BB: Cardiopulmonary resuscitation in a pediatric ICU. *Crit Care Med* 14:275, 1986.
11. O'Rourke PP: Outcome of children who are apneic and pulseless in the emergency room. *Crit Care Med* 14:466, 1986.

Basic Life Support

Basic life support includes epidemiology, prevention, recognition of distress and/or arrest, actions for survival, cardiopulmonary resuscitation, airway obstruction management, and access to emergency medical services. It is assumed that prior to taking an ALS course, the student will have learned the principles and mastered the concepts and skills of BLS. However, since BLS for infants and small children is different in many respects from that for adults and since ALS is not possible without skill in the techniques of BLS, these differences and techniques will be reviewed in this chapter.

I. Epidemiology of Cardiopulmonary Arrest

Childhood is the healthiest period of life; beyond the first month death rates are lower in childhood than at any subsequent time. Nonetheless, approximately 40,000 infants under 1 year of age and 16,000 children between the ages 1 and 14 years die annually in the United States.[1]

A. Age

A review of several studies[2–12] suggests that cardiopulmonary resuscitation is most frequently required in the very young. Over half the patients are less than 1 year of age, and within that age group, the majority are less than 4 months old.

B. Predisposing Factors

Cardiac arrest in the pediatric age group is rarely primarily of cardiac origin; more commonly, it results from hypoxemia secondary to a respiratory or circulatory cause. Major events that may necessitate resuscitation are numerous and include 1) injuries, 2) suffocation caused by a foreign body, i.e., toys, foods, plastic covers, etc., 3) smoke inhalation, 4) sudden infant death syndrome (SIDS), and 5) infections, especially of the respiratory tract. Injuries are the leading cause of pediatric deaths in the United States and represent approximately 44% of deaths in children between the ages of 1 and 14 years. Of these, 45% involve motor vehicles, 17% drowning, and 21% burns, firearms, and poisoning.[13]

C. Outcome

In the pediatric age group, cardiac arrest is most frequently the end result of a long period of hypoxemia secondary to inadequate oxygenation, ventilation, or circulation (shock), which may be initiated by many predisposing conditions. Once cardiac arrest occurs, the outcome of resuscitative attempts is poor. This is not surprising since the prolonged period of hypoxemia or shock causes damage to many organs, including the brain. Outcome following intervention for respiratory arrest is considerably better.

Gillis, et al.,[12] reviewed in-hospital resuscitations and found a 6-month survival of 17%; 44% of children survived following resuscitation from respiratory arrest, but only 9% following cardiac arrest. Friesen, et al.,[5] reviewed all pediatric cardiac arrests in Manitoba. Cardiac output was restored in 36% of the children, but only 9% ultimately survived; one half of the survivors were neurologically normal while the other half suffered major neurologic damage. Respiratory arrest was associated with a better survival (40%) than cardiac arrest (2%). O'Rourke[8] reviewed a group of out-of-hospital cardiac arrest victims who were successfully resuscitated and admitted to an intensive care unit; only 21% survived to discharge and all had a poor neurologic outcome.

II. Prevention

The diverse, but often preventable, causes of cardiopulmonary arrest in children, coupled with the poor outcome once cardiac arrest has taken place, have implications for community strategies for dealing with the problem. The preventable nature of many of the causes suggests that special attention must be given to public education programs that emphasize prevention. An environment should be created that is safe and protective without suppressing the child's intellectual curiosity and need for exploration and discovery. Children should be taught respect for matches and fires, and the use of smoke detectors should be encouraged.[14] Toys given to toddlers should be carefully examined for small parts that can be aspirated into the airway.[15] Beads, small toys, marbles, and peanuts must be kept away from infants and preschool children. The use of age-appropriate restraints and infant car seats have been shown to be life-saving.[16] Children should be taught to swim, and water safety programs should be provided.[17]

The poor outcome of cardiac resuscitation should lead to an educational emphasis, for both the lay and the professional public, of the recognition and potential danger of respiratory difficulty in infants and children. Airway management and ventilation should be emphasized as the most important maneuvers in the resuscitation effort. Healthcare providers should be optimally trained to recognize pediatric emergencies and properly equipped to care for them. There is evidence that this is not currently the case.[18,19]

III. The Sequence of Cardiopulmonary Resuscitation: The ABC's of CPR

Cardiopulmonary resuscitation consists of a series of maneuvers by which oxygenated blood flow to the brain and other vital organs can be maintained.[20] In basic life support, CPR requires skills, but no adjuncts, and can be performed in most locations and under most circumstances, speed and skill being the two most crucial factors for success.

A. AIRWAY

1. Assessment: Determine Unresponsiveness or Respiratory Difficulty

The rescuer must quickly assess the extent of any injury or respiratory difficulty and determine whether the child is conscious. Unconsciousness is determined by gently shaking the victim to elicit a response. If the child has sustained head or neck trauma, special care must be taken to avoid injury to the spinal cord. If a child is struggling to breathe but is conscious, the child should be transported as rapidly as possible to an ALS facility. Children will often find the best position in which to keep a partially obstructed airway open and should therefore be allowed to maintain the position affording them the greatest comfort.

2. Call for Help

After determining unresponsiveness or respiratory difficulty, the rescuer should call out for help. If the rescuer is alone and the child is not breathing, CPR should be performed for 1 minute *before* activating EMS.

3. Position the Victim

For CPR to be effective, the victim must be supine, on a firm, flat surface. Great care must be taken in moving the child if head or neck injury is suspected; manual in-line cervical stabilization *must* be maintained until cervical spine injury is excluded or the neck is properly immobilized. The child must be turned as a unit, with firm support of the head and neck so that the head does not roll, twist, or tilt backward or forward.

4. Open the Airway

During unconsciousness, muscle relaxation causes airway obstruction by passive posterior displacement of the tongue.[21] The airway should be opened by head-tilt/chin-lift or, when neck injury is suspected, by the jaw-thrust maneuver. If a child is having respiratory difficulty but is conscious, time should not be wasted on attempting to open the airway; the child should be transported to an ALS facility as rapidly as possible.

Head-Tilt/Chin-Lift: The rescuer should place the hand closest to the child's head on the forehead and tilt

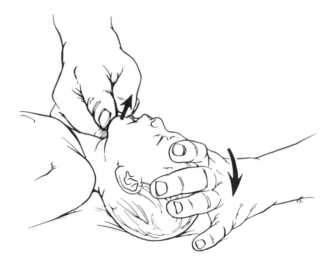

Figure 2.1. Head-tilt/chin-lift.

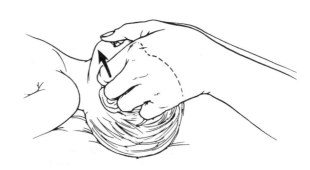

Figure 2.2. Jaw-thrust.

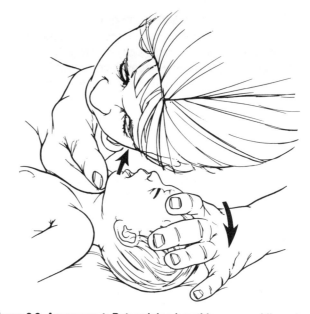

Figure 2.3. Assessment: Determining breathlessness while maintaining head-tilt/chin-lift — *look, listen, feel.*

the head back gently into a "sniffing" or neutral position in an infant, and slightly further back in a child (Figure 2.1). The fingers, but not the thumb, of the rescuer's other hand should be placed under the bony part of the lower jaw at the chin; and the chin should be lifted upward. Care must be taken not to close the mouth or to push on the soft tissues under the chin, so as not to obstruct the airway. If neck injury is suspected, head-tilt should be avoided and the airway should be opened by jaw-thrust without head-tilt.

Jaw-Thrust: The rescuer should place two or three fingers under each side of the lower jaw at its angle and lift the jaw upward (Figure 2.2). The rescuer's elbows should rest on the surface on which the victim is lying. Jaw-thrust may be accompanied by slight head-tilt when jaw-thrust alone does not open the airway. Jaw-thrust, without head-tilt, is the safest technique for opening the airway when neck injury is suspected.

B. BREATHING

5. Assessment: Determine Whether the Victim Is Breathing

If it is unclear whether the victim is breathing, the rescuer should open the airway and, while maintaining patency, place his or her ear close to the victim's mouth and nose, watch for the rise and fall of the chest and abdomen, listen for exhaled air, and feel for exhaled air flow (Figure 2.3). If the child is breathing or resumes breathing, patency of the airway must be maintained. If the victim is not breathing, the rescuer must administer rescue breathing.

6. Rescue Breathing

While the airway is kept open, the rescuer should inhale and make a seal with his or her mouth and the victim's mouth, or mouth and nose. If the victim is an infant, the seal should be made with the victim's mouth and nose. If the victim is a large infant or a child, the victim's nose should be pinched with the thumb and forefingers of the rescuer's hand that is maintaining head-tilt, and a mouth-to-mouth seal should be made (Figure 2.4). *Two slow* breaths (1–1.5 sec/breath) should be delivered, with a pause between them to allow the rescuer to take a breath. Because of a wide variation in sizes of victims, it is impossible to make precise recommendations on the pressure or volume of ventilations. The critical things to remember are that:

1. ventilation is the most important rescue maneuver in a nonbreathing infant or child victim;
2. an appropriate volume of air is one that causes the chest to rise;
3. the small airways of the infant or child may result in a high resistance to air flow; and
4. by giving breaths slowly, an adequate volume will be provided at the lowest possible pressure, thereby avoiding gastric distention.[22,23]

If air enters freely and the chest rises, the airway is clear. If air does not enter freely (i.e., the chest does not rise), the airway is obstructed. Since improper opening of the airway is the most common cause of obstruction, head-tilt/chin-lift should be readjusted. If the airway remains obstructed, obstruction by a foreign body must be suspected.

C. CIRCULATION

7. Assessment: Check the Pulse

Ineffective or absent cardiac contractions are recognized by the absence of a pulse in a large central artery. In children over 1 year of age, the carotid is the most

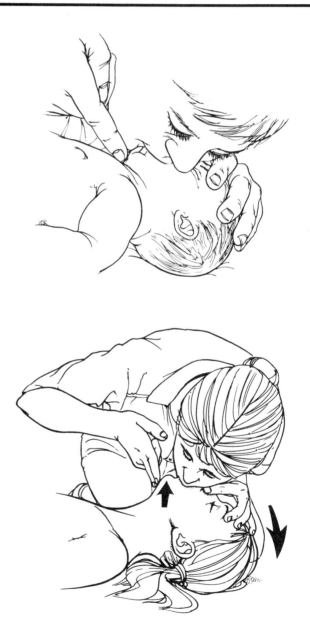

Figure 2.4. Administering rescue breathing. Top: Mouth-to-mouth-and-nose seal (infant). Bottom: Mouth-to-mouth-seal (child).

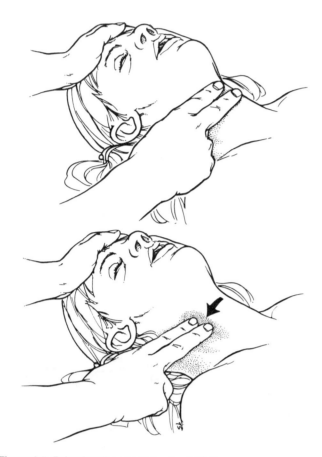

Figure 2.5. Palpating the carotid pulse (child).

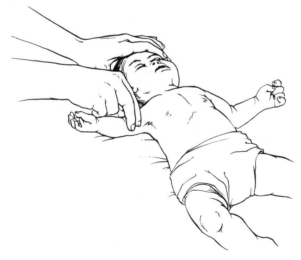

Figure 2.6. Palpating the brachial pulse (infant).

accessible central artery. In infants under 1 year of age, the short chubby neck makes the carotid artery difficult to palpate, and therefore, the brachial or femoral arteries are recommended. (For the sake of simplicity, only the brachial location is taught to lay rescuers.) Precordial activity represents an impulse rather than a pulse, and its absence does not correlate with absent cardiac activity.[24]

The carotid artery lies on the side of the neck between the trachea and the strap muscles. To feel it the rescuer locates the victim's Adam's apple with two or three fingers of one hand while maintaining head-tilt with the other hand on the forehead. The fingers are then slid into the groove between the trachea and the neck muscles on the side nearest the rescuer, and the artery is gently palpated (Figure 2.5).

The brachial pulse is located on the inside of the upper arm, between elbow and shoulder. With the rescuer's thumb on the outside of the arm, the index and middle fingers are pressed gently until the pulse is felt (Figure 2.6).

If a pulse is present but spontaneous breathing is absent, ventilations are continued at a rate of 20 breaths/min for an infant and 15 breaths/min for a child. If a pulse is not palpable, chest compressions must be initiated and coordinated with ventilations.

8. Activate the Emergency Medical Services (EMS) System

If a second rescuer is present or arrives to help, one rescuer should activate the Emergency Medical Services (EMS) system by calling the local emergency number (in many communities, 911). If no help is forthcoming, the decision whether to leave the victim in order to telephone is a difficult one, affected by a number of variables, including the probability of someone else arriving on the scene. If a rescuer is alone, CPR should be performed for 1 minute *before* activating the EMS system. If the rescuer is unable to activate the EMS system, the only option is to continue CPR.

The rescuer calling the EMS system should give the following information:

1. Location of the emergency (address, names of streets or landmarks).
2. Phone number from which the call is being made.
3. What happened (i.e., auto accident, drowning, etc.).
4. Number of victims.
5. Condition of the victim(s).
6. Nature of the aid being given.
7. Any other information requested.

To assure that the person taking the information gets all he or she needs in order to respond effectively and efficiently, *the caller should hang up last.*

9. Perform Chest Compressions

Since its introduction in 1960,[25] the technique of external chest compressions has been accepted as a method of maintaining a minimal cardiac output capable of sustaining the vital organs. The mechanism by which blood circulates during chest compressions, especially in infants and children, is a matter of controversy.[26–29] The "thoracic pump" theory holds that blood circulates as a result of a change in intrathoracic vs. extrathoracic pressures during compressions. According to the "cardiac pump" theory, circulation takes place as a result of direct compression of

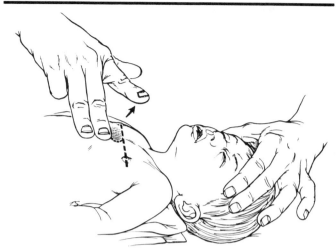

Figure 2.7. Locating the correct position for the fingers in chest compressions in the infant.

the heart. Direct heart compression may be the more important mechanism in the pediatric age group.[30,31]

Indications for performing chest compressions are: 1) asystole, as evidenced by an absent pulse, and 2) any other non-perfusing rhythm (e.g., pulseless ventricular tachycardia, ventricular fibrillation).

For optimal compressions, the child must be in a horizontal, supine position on a hard surface, which for an infant can be the palm of the rescuer's hand supporting the back. This maneuver also raises the shoulders, which allows the infant's head to tilt back, thus maintaining airway patency.

In the Infant: Recent evidence has shown that the heart in an infant is lower in relation to external chest landmarks than was previously thought.[32–34] In the following recommendations, therefore, the area of compression is lower than in previous standards (Figure 2.7).

1. A line is imagined between the nipples over the sternum (breastbone) — the intermammary line.
2. The index finger of the hand farthest from the infant's head is placed just under the intermammary line where it intersects the sternum. The area of compression is approximately one finger's width, or less, *below* this intersection, at the location of the middle and ring fingers; the rescuer must take care not to compress the xiphoid.
3. Using two or three fingers, the sternum is compressed to a depth of 0.5–1 inch (1.3–2.5 cm) at a rate of at least 100 times/min.
4. At the end of each compression, pressure is released and, without lifting the fingers off, the sternum is allowed to come to its normal position. A smooth compress–release rhythm, i.e., without jerky movements, should be developed in which the time allotted to each phase of the cycle is equal.

In the Child: At older than approximately 1 year of age, a patient is considered a child for purposes of BLS.

1. With the middle and index fingers of the hand nearest the victim's feet, the lower margin of the victim's rib cage is located on the side next to the rescuer (Figure 2.8).
2. The margin of the rib cage is followed with the middle finger to the notch where the ribs and sternum meet.
3. With the middle finger on this notch, the index finger is placed next to the middle finger.
4. The heel of the same hand is placed next to the previous location of the index finger, with the long axis of the heel parallel to that of the sternum.
5. The sternum is compressed with one hand to a depth of 1 to 1.5 inches (2.5–3.8 cm) at a rate of 80–100 times/min. The fingers should be kept off the ribs.
6. The compressions should be smooth, not jerky. The chest should be allowed to return to its resting position after each compression, but the hand should not be lifted off the chest. Each compression and relaxation phase should be of equal time.
7. If the child is large or above the age of approximately 8 years, the method described for adults should be used.

10. Coordinate Compressions and Breathing

External chest compressions must always be accompanied by ventilations. At the end of every fifth compression a pause (1–1.5 seconds) should be allowed for ventilation. In the infant and child a 5:1 compression:ventilation ratio is maintained for both one and two rescuers. (The two-rescuer technique should be used only by healthcare providers.) The victim should be reassessed after 10 cycles of compressions and ventilations (approximately 1 minute) and every few minutes thereafter.

Coordination of compressions and ventilations by a sin-

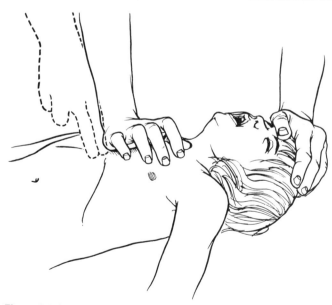

Figure 2.8. Locating the correct position for the hand in chest compressions in the child.

Table 2.1. Summary of BLS Maneuvers in Infants and Children.

	Infant	Child
AIRWAY	Head-tilt/chin-lift Jaw-thrust	Head-tilt/chin-lift Jaw-thrust
BREATHING		
Initial	Two breaths at 1.0–1.5 sec/breath	Two breaths at 1.0–1.5 sec/breath
Subsequent	20 breaths/minute	15 breaths/minute
CIRCULATION		
Pulse check	Brachial/femoral	Carotid
Compression area	Lower third of sternum	Lower third of sternum
Compressed with	2–3 fingers	Heel of one hand
Depth	0.5–1.0 inch (approx.)	1.0–1.5 inch (approx.)
Rate	At least 100/minute	80–100/minute
Compression: ventilation ratio	5:1 (pause for ventilation)	5:1 (pause for ventilation)
FOREIGN BODY AIRWAY OBSTRUCTION	Back blows/chest thrusts	Heimlich maneuver

gle rescuer involves compromises. In infants, after the initial two ventilations, airway patency must be maintained by head-tilt alone. In general this is satisfactory, but the chest should be carefully observed to make sure it rises with each rescue breath. If the airway were to be opened after each five compressions by head-tilt/chin-lift using the hand performing compressions, the total number of compressions would be drastically reduced. In children, head-tilt alone may be inadequate to maintain airway patency. The head-tilt/chin-lift maneuver is therefore performed with each ventilation. The compromise here is that the hand performing the compressions is moved back to the chest without going through the full, correct procedure for finding the landmark each time. If the landmarks were correctly located after each ventilation, the total number of compressions would be inadequate.

A summary of BLS maneuvers in infants and children is presented in Table 2.1.

IV. Airway Obstruction Management

More than 90% of deaths from aspirations of foreign bodies in the pediatric age group occur in children younger than 5 years of age, and 65% involve infants. Aspirated materials include food (i.e., hot dogs, round candies, nuts, grapes) and other small objects.[35] Foreign body airway obstruction should be suspected in infants and children experiencing the sudden onset of respiratory distress associated with coughing, gagging, and stridor.

Signs and symptoms of airway obstruction may also be due to infections that can cause airway swelling, such as epiglottitis and croup. Children with an infectious cause of airway obstruction need prompt attention in an ALS facility, and time should not be wasted in a futile and dangerous attempt to relieve their obstruction.

Attempts at clearing the airway should be considered for 1) the child in whom the aspiration of a foreign body is

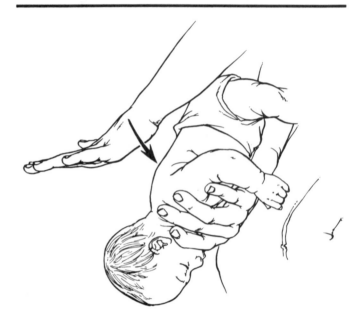

Figure 2.9. Positioning an infant for back blows.

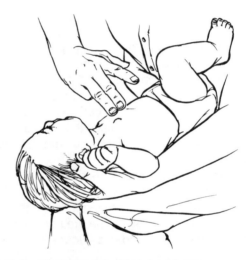

Figure 2.10. Positioning an infant for chest thrusts.

witnessed or strongly suspected, and 2) the unconscious, nonbreathing child whose airway remains obstructed despite the usual maneuvers to open it. In a witnessed or seriously suspected foreign body aspiration, the rescuer should encourage the child to persist with spontaneous coughing and breathing efforts as long as the cough is forceful. *Relief of the obstruction should be attempted only if the cough becomes ineffective and/or there is increased respiratory difficulty accompanied by stridor.*

The optimal method for relief of foreign body obstruction remains a matter of controversy, and further data are needed to distinguish opinions and personal experiences from objective facts. If the victim is a child, the Heimlich maneuver, a series of subdiaphragmatic abdominal thrusts, is recommended.[36–39] This maneuver, by increasing intrathoracic pressure, creates an artificial cough that forces air and, it is hoped, the foreign body out of the airway. Six to 10 thrusts are repeated in rapid sequence until the foreign body is expelled.

Because of concern for potential intraabdominal injury resulting from the Heimlich maneuver in infants, a combination of back blows and chest thrusts is recommended for the relief of foreign body airway obstruction in this age group.[40]

Following maneuvers to relieve an obstructed airway, the airway is opened using head-tilt/chin-lift; if spontaneous breathing is absent, rescue breathing is performed. If the chest does not rise, the head is repositioned, the airway is opened, and rescue breathing is again attempted. If rescue breathing is still unsuccessful (i.e., the chest does not rise), maneuvers to relieve a foreign body airway obstruction should be repeated.

A. The Infant — Back Blows and Chest Thrusts

The infant is straddled over the rescuer's arm, with the head lower than the trunk, and the head is supported by firmly holding the jaw. For additional support, the rescuer rests his or her forearm on the thigh (Figure 2.9). Four

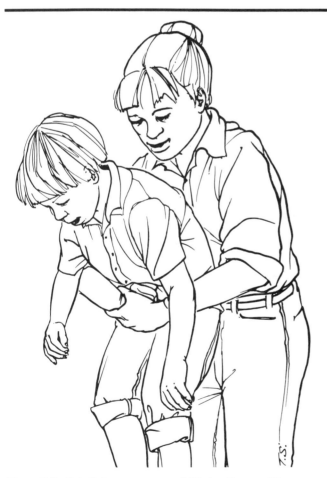

Figure 2.11. Heimlich maneuver — child standing or sitting (conscious).

back blows are forcefully given with the heel of the hand between the infant's shoulder blades. After delivering the back blows, the rescuer places his or her free hand on the infant's back so that the infant is sandwiched between the two hands, one supporting the neck, jaw, and chest, while the other supports the back. With continuing support to the head and neck, the infant is turned and placed on the thigh with the head lower than the trunk, and four chest thrusts are performed in the same location as chest compressions but at a slower rate (Figure 2.10).

Rescuers whose hands are small may find it difficult to perform the back blows and chest thrusts in the manner described above, especially if the infant is large. An alternate method is to lay the infant face down on the rescuer's lap, with the head lower than the trunk, and firmly supported. After the four back blows have been given, the infant is turned as a unit to the supine position and four chest thrusts are performed.

B. The Child — Subdiaphragmatic Abdominal Thrusts (Heimlich Maneuver)

1. Heimlich Maneuver With Victim Standing or Sitting (Conscious)

The rescuer stands behind the victim and wraps his/her arms around the victim's waist, with one hand made into a fist (Figure 2.11). The thumb side of the fist should rest against the victim's abdomen, in the midline slightly above the navel and well below the tip of the xiphoid process. The fist is grasped by the other hand and pressed into the victim's abdomen with a quick upward thrust. The rescuer's hands should not be touching the xiphoid process or the lower margin of the rib cage so as not to damage the internal organs.[41,42] Each thrust should be a separate and distinct movement. The series is continued until the foreign body is expelled or 10 thrusts are completed.

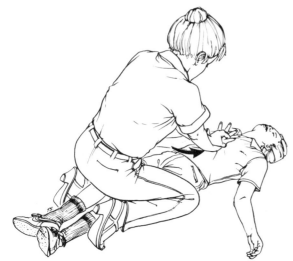

Figure 2.12. Heimlich maneuver — child lying (unconscious).

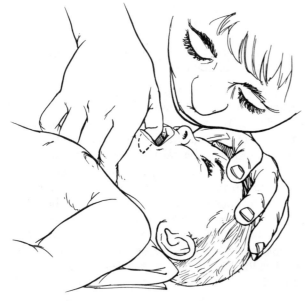

Figure 2.13. Tongue–jaw lift.

2. Heimlich Maneuver With Victim Lying (Unconscious)

The rescuer positions the child face up on his/her back and kneels at the child's feet, if on the floor, or stands at the child's feet, if the victim is on a table (Figure 2.12). The astride position may be used if the child is large. The rescuer places the heel of one hand on the child's abdomen in the midline slightly above the navel and well below the rib cage. The other hand is placed on top of the first and pressed into the abdomen with a quick upward thrust. A series (6–10) of upward thrusts is performed, each thrust being a separate and distinct movement. Care should be exercised to direct each thrust upward in the midline, not to either side of the abdomen.

C. Manual Removal of Foreign Bodies

Blind finger sweeps of the throat for removing foreign bodies should be avoided in infants and children since the foreign body may be pushed back into the airway and cause further obstruction. In the unconscious, nonbreathing victim, following the chest or subdiaphragmatic thrusts, the victim's mouth should be opened by grasping both the tongue and the lower jaw between the thumb and finger and lifting (tongue–jaw lift) (Figure 2.13). This action draws the tongue away from the back of the throat and may itself partially relieve the obstruction. If the foreign body is visualized, it should be removed.

V. Mouth-to-Mask Ventilation and Cricoid Pressure

Healthcare providers must learn the techniques of mouth-to-mask ventilation and cricoid pressure as part of their basic life support training. These techniques offer some advantages in resuscitation situations, but they both require two rescuers for proper performance. *Note:* The Centers for Disease Control recommend that, though it has not been shown that HIV is transmitted via saliva, the need for mouth-to-*mouth* resuscitation should be reduced as much as possible by making masks with one-way valves, resuscitation bags, or other ventilation devices available for use in all areas in which the need for resuscitation is predictable.[43]

Face masks and their sizes are described in Chapter 3, Section III, Part B. The technique should be as follows:

1. Ventilator: Open the airway by head-tilt. Apply the rim of the mask first between the victim's lower lip and the chin, thus retracting the lower lip to keep the mouth open. Once the mask is on the face of the victim, clamp it with both thumbs on the sides of the mask to provide a seal between the face and the mask. The index, middle, and ring fingers should grasp the lower jaw just above the angles of the mandible and apply pressure upward. The airway is maintained open by a combination of head-tilt/jaw-thrust.
2. Ventilate through the mouthpiece according to the recommendations for two-rescuer CPR (see Appendix A). A tight seal is essential to prevent loss of volume during ventilations.

Cricoid pressure (the Sellick maneuver) is described, including technique, in Chapter 3, Section III, Part B.

VI. Sequences for Specific Rescue Situation

There is an optimum sequence of actions for each of the most common rescue situations. These sequences are described in detail in Appendix A.

References

1. NCHS Monthly Vital Statistics Report. 32:16, 1984.
2. Ehrlich R, Emmett SM, Rodgiguez-Torres R: Pediatric cardiac resuscitation team: A 6 year study. *J Peds* 84:152, 1974.
3. Ludwig S, Kettrick RG, Parker M: Pediatric cardiopulmonary resuscitation. A review of 130 cases. *Clin Pediatr* 23:71, 1984.
4. DeBard ML: Cardiopulmonary resuscitation: Analysis of six years' experience and review of the literature. *Ann Emerg Med* 10:408, 1981.
5. Friesen RM, Duncan P, Tweed WA, et al: Appraisal of pediatric cardiopulmonary resuscitation. *Can Med Assoc J* 126:1055, 1982.
6. Eisenberg M, Bergner L, Hallstrom A: Epidemiology of cardiac arrest and resuscitation in children. *Ann Emerg Med* 12:672, 1983.
7. Lewis JK, Minter MG, Eshelman SJ, et al: Outcome of pediatric resuscitation. *Ann Emerg Med* 12:297, 1983.
8. O'Rourke PP: Outcome of children who are apneic and pulseless in the emergency room. *Crit Care Med* 14:466, 1986.
9. Nichols DG, Kettrick RG, Swedlow DB, et al: Factors influencing outcome of cardiopulmonary arrest in children (abstract). *Crit Care Med* 12:287, 1984.
10. Torphy DE, Minter MG, Thompson BM: Cardiorespiratory arrest and resuscitation of children. *Am J Dis Child* 138:1099, 1984.
11. Rosenberg NM: Pediatric cardiopulmonary arrest in the emergency department. *Am J Emerg Med* 2:497, 1984.
12. Gillis J, Dickson D, Rieder M, et al: Results of inpatient pediatric resuscitation. *Crit Care Med* 14:469, 1986.
13. Statistical Resources Branch, Division of Vital Statistics: *Final Mortality Statistics 1981.* Hyattsville, Md., National Center for Health Statistics, 1984.
14. *Fire in the United States,* ed 4. Washington, D.C., Federal Emergency Management Agency, 1983, pp 25–26.
15. Baker SP, Fisher RS: Childhood asphyxiation by choking or suffocation. *JAMA* 244:1343, 1980.
16. Decker MD, Dewey J, Hutcheson RH, et al: The use and efficacy of child restraint devices. The Tennessee experience, 1982 and 1983. *JAMA* 252:2571, 1984.
17. Pearn J, Nixon J: Prevention of childhood drowning accidents. *Med J Aust* 1:616, 1977.
18. Seidel JS, Hornbein M, Yoshiyama K, et al: Emergency Medical Services and the pediatric patient: Are the needs being met? *Pediatrics* 73:769, 1984.
19. Seidel JS: Emergency Medical Services and the pediatric patient: Are the needs being met? II. Training and equipping Emergency Medical Services providers for pediatric emergencies. *Pediatrics* 78:808, 1986.
20. Standards and Guidelines for Cardiopulmonary Resuscitation (CPR) and Emergency Cardiac Care (ECC). *JAMA* 255:2954, 1986.
21. Ruben HM, Elam JO, Ruben AM, et al: Investigation of upper airway problems in resuscitation. 1. Studies of pharyngeal x-rays and performance of laymen. *Anesthesiology* 22:271, 1961.
22. Melker RJ: Asynchronous and other alternative methods of ventilation during CPR. *Ann Emerg Med* 13:758, 1984.
23. Melker RJ, Banner MJ: Ventilation during CPR: Two rescuer standards reappraised. *Ann Emerg Med* 14:397, 1985.
24. Cavallaro DL, Melker RJ: Comparison of two techniques for detecting cardiac activity in infants. *Crit Care Med* 11:189, 1983.
25. Kouwenhoven WB, Jude JR, Knickerbocker GG: Closed chest cardiac massage. *JAMA* 173:1064, 1960.
26. Babbs CF: New versus old theories of blood flow during CPR. *Crit Care Med* 8:191, 1980.
27. Rudikoff MT, Maughan WC, Effron M, et al: Mechanism of blood flow during cardiopulmonary resuscitation. *Circulation* 61:345, 1980.
28. Werner JA, Greene HL, Janko CL, et al: Visualization of cardiac valve motion in man during external chest compression using two-dimensional echocardiography. Implications regarding the mechanism of blood flow. *Circulation* 63:1417, 1981.
29. Maier GW, Tyson GS Jr, Olsen CO, et al: The physiology of external cardiac massage: High-impulse cardiopulmonary resuscitation. *Circulation* 70:86, 1984.
30. Koehler RC, Michael JR, Guerci AD, et al: Beneficial effect of epinephrine infusion on cerebral and myocardial blood flows during CPR. *Ann Emerg Med* 14:744, 1985.
31. Schleien CL, Dean JM, Koehler RC, et al: Effect of epinephrine on cerebral and myocardial perfusion in an infant animal preparation of cardiopulmonary resuscitation. *Circulation* 73:809, 1986.
32. Phillips GW, Zideman DA: Relation of infant heart to sternum: Its significance in cardiopulmonary resuscitation. *Lancet* 1:1024, 1986.
33. Orlowski J: Optimum position for external cardiac compression in infants and young children. *Ann Emerg Med* 15:667, 1986.
34. Finholt DA, Kettrick RG, Wagner HR, et al: The heart is under the lower third of the sternum. Implications for external cardiac massage. *Am J Dis Child* 140:646, 1986.
35. Harris CS, Baker SP, Smith GA, et al: Childhood asphyxiation by food. A national analysis and overview. *JAMA* 251:2231, 1984.
36. Day RL, Crelin ES, Dubois AB: Choking: The Heimlich abdominal thrust vs. back blows. An approach to measurement of inertial and aerodynamic forces. *Pediatrics* 70:113, 1982.
37. Eigen H: Treatment of choking. *Pediatrics* 71:300, 1983.
38. Day RL: Differing opinions on the emergency treatment of choking. *Pediatrics* 71:976, 1983.
39. Heimlich HJ: A life-saving maneuver to prevent food choking. *JAMA* 234:398, 1975.
40. Standards and Guidelines for Cardiopulmonary Resuscitation (CPR) and Emergency Cardiac Care (ECC) *JAMA* 244:475, 1980.
41. Visintine RE, Baick CH: Ruptured stomach after Heimlich maneuver. *JAMA* 234:415, 1975.
42. Palmer E: The Heimlich maneuver misused. *Current Prescribing* 5:45, 1979.
43. Centers for Disease Control: Recommendations for prevention of HIV transmission in health-care settings. MMWR 36 (suppl):2, 1987.

Pediatric Airway Management

The respiratory system delivers oxygen to the blood and eliminates carbon dioxide. Failure of this system is common in infants and children, and treatment decisions must be made quickly to avert a downhill progression from respiratory distress to respiratory failure and, finally, cardiopulmonary arrest. Respiratory difficulties are an important cause of both in- and out-of-hospital pediatric cardiopulmonary arrest;[1,2] in hospitalized children they are approximately twice as common as other causes.[2-4] Once cardiac arrest occurs, outcome is poor.[5,6] Therefore, early recognition and management of airway problems are major facets of pediatric advanced life support.

This chapter is a review of the wide variety of adjuncts used in airway management and of the priorities of assessment and treatment. This knowledge must be mastered and blended into the overall management of the patient.

I. Anatomic and Physiologic Considerations

The pediatric airway differs from that of the adult in several important anatomic and physiologic ways.[7] Anatomic differences of the upper airway include the following: 1) The larynx is relatively cephalad in position; 2) the epiglottis is "U" shaped and protrudes into the pharynx; 3) the vocal cords are short and concave; and 4) in infants and children less than 8 years of age the narrowest portion of the airway is at the cricoid cartilage below the cords, in contrast to older children and adults, in whom the narrowest portion is at the vocal cords. These anatomic differences have the following important practical consequences:

1. It is difficult to create a single, clear, visual plane from the mouth through the pharynx to the glottis for laryngoscopy or endotracheal intubation.
2. Endotracheal tube size must be selected based on the size of the cricoid ring rather than the glottic opening.

The lower airways are smaller and their supporting cartilage less developed in the infant and young child than in the adult; therefore, they can easily become obstructed by mucus, blood, pus, edema, or active constriction. Extrinsic obstruction (e.g., a vascular ring or tumor) may also occur. Airway obstruction results in increased airway resistance, the latter being inversely proportional to the 4th power of the radius (Figure 3.1). Even a minor reduction in the already small diameter of the pediatric airway results in a large reduction in the cross-sectional area.

The ribs and sternum normally support the lung and help it remain expanded, while the intercostal muscles and diaphragm alter intrathoracic pressure and volume, leading to movement of air. In the young victim, the ribs are pliable and fail to support the lung, leading to paradoxical movement (sternal and intercostal retractions) during active inspiration, rather than expansion of the lung. In addition, tidal volume in the pediatric patient is much more dependent on diaphragmatic function and movement. When diaphragmatic movement is impeded by pressure from above (pulmonary hyperinflation, e.g., asthma) or from below (gastric or abdominal distension), effective respiration is compromised since the chest wall cannot compensate.

The pediatric patient is further compromised by a high metabolic rate (oxygen consumption is 6–8 mL/kg/min in a child compared to 3–4 mL/kg/min in an adult). With onset of apnea or inadequate alveolar ventilation, hypoxemia occurs more rapidly in the child.

An illness leading to respiratory distress or failure may exacerbate hypoxemia by several mechanisms:

1. The disease process decreases lung compliance (making the lungs stiffer) and increases work of breathing and, therefore, metabolic (oxygen consuming) demand.
2. The disease process directly interferes with exchange of oxygen or carbon dioxide.
3. Mismatching of ventilation and pulmonary perfusion causes shunting of pulmonary blood through the lung so that hypoxemia and, to a lesser extent, hypercapnia occur.

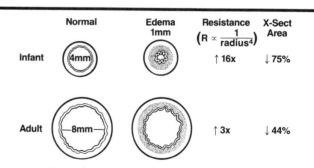

Figure 3.1. Effects of edema on airway resistance in the infant vs. the adult. Normal airways are represented on the left; edematous airways (1 mm circumferential edema), on the right. Resistance to flow is inversely proportional to the radius of the lumen to the fourth power for laminar flow, and the fifth power for turbulent flow. The net result is a 75% decrease in cross-sectional area and a 16-fold increase in resistance in the infant vs. 44% and 3-fold respectively in the adult. (From Coté CJ, Todres ID: The pediatric airway, in Ryan JF, Todres ID, Coté CJ, Goudsouzian N [eds]: *A Practice of Anesthesia for Infants and Children.* New York, Grune & Stratton, Inc., 1986, p. 39.)

Table 3.1. The Goals and Equipment/Techniques of Airway Therapy

Goal: Airway Patency	Goal: Oxygenation	Goal: Ventilation	Goal: Airway Protection
Head and jaw position	Oxygen	Mask	Suction devices
Oropharyngeal airway	Nasal cannula	Cricoid pressure	Cricoid pressure
Nasopharyngeal airway	Nasal catheter*	Endotracheal airway	Endotracheal airway
Suction devices	Oxygen hood	Esophageal obturator airway*	Esophageal obturator airway*
Endotracheal airway	Oxygen tent	Self-inflating bag–valve ventilating device	
Esophageal obturator airway*	Oxygen mask	Anesthesia ventilating system	
Cricothyrotomy	Face tent	Oxygen-powered breathing device*	
	Self-inflating bag–valve ventilating device	Cricothyrotomy and transtracheal catheter ventilation*	
	Anesthesia ventilating system		
	Continuous positive airway pressure (CPAP)		
	Positive end-expiratory pressure (PEEP)		
	Oxygen-powered breathing device*		
	Cricothyrotomy and transtracheal catheter ventilation*		

*Not recommended for use in infants and children.

Compromise of ventilatory function may also result from depression of central control of ventilation by hypoxemia, hypothermia, medications, metabolic derangements (e.g., hypoglycemia), or head trauma. Apnea is relatively common in ill infants and head-injured children, so respiratory activity should be carefully monitored. Fortunately, cervical spine injuries are relatively uncommon in infants and children. However, high spinal injury (i.e., C4 and above) may cause apnea by disrupting the innervation of the diaphragm.

II. Airway Adjuncts for the Spontaneously Breathing Patient in Respiratory Distress

A. General Principles

The goals of emergency airway therapy are to *anticipate* and *recognize* respiratory problems and support or supplant those functions that are compromised or lost (Table 3.1). In an emergency, the etiology of the respiratory dysfunction may not always be clear, or necessary, in order to initiate some or all of the steps of emergency airway management.

The infant or child with signs of acute respiratory distress (see Chapter 1) should be immediately provided with humidified oxygen in the highest concentration available. Humidification is essential to prevent obstruction of the infant's or child's small airway with dried secretions. Heated humidification systems are preferable to cool mist systems,

which can produce hypothermia in the small victim.

In patients with chronic respiratory insufficiency (elevated $PaCO_2$) administration of high concentrations of oxygen may abolish respiratory drive, with disastrous consequences, unless the patient is carefully monitored. Children at risk include those with advanced cystic fibrosis and bronchopulmonary dysplasia. In the vast majority of acute respiratory emergencies, high FiO_2 can be delivered without acute harmful effects.

Alert children usually assume an optimal position for airway patency and ease of ventilation and should be allowed to do so. A child should not be forced to lay supine since anxiety will add to the child's oxygen consumption and may increase the respiratory distress. Children who are *alert* should be allowed to remain with their parents and be slowly introduced to airway equipment, including oxygen. For example, a child who is upset by an oxygen mask may be calmed by having the parent blow a stream of humidified oxygen toward the child's mouth and nose.

If the child is somnolent or unconscious, the airway may be obstructed by a combination of flexion of the head and flaccidity of the jaw and tongue, which falls against the posterior wall of the pharynx. In this setting noninvasive methods of opening the airway (see Chapter 2) should precede the use of adjuncts. Suctioning secretions, mucus, or blood from the oro- and nasopharynx may be sufficient to achieve a clear airway.

If, despite the administration of oxygen and a patent airway, ventilation is inadequate (as judged by insufficient chest movement and inadequate breath sounds), assisted ventilation should be provided. Assisted ventilation in the patient with respiratory failure must not await the placement of an endotracheal tube. In the vast majority of respiratory emergencies, infants and children can be successfully ventilated with a bag–valve–mask device, even when airway obstruction from conditions such as acute epiglottitis produces respiratory failure.[8] Gentle positive-pressure breaths given by a bag–valve–mask device are carefully timed to augment the child's inspiratory efforts. Breaths not coordinated with the child's efforts may be ineffective and cause coughing, retching, and gastric distension.

B. Oxygen Delivery Systems[9]

Oxygen delivery systems can be divided into "low-flow" and "high-flow" systems. A low-flow system is one in which the gas flow is insufficient to meet all inspiratory flow requirements and, therefore, air is entrained. A high-flow system is one in which the flow rate and reservoir capacity are adequate to provide the total inspired flow rate of the patient. Although low-flow systems are thought of as low oxygen delivery systems, the oxygen concentration delivered depends on the patient's minute ventilation and can vary from .23 to .90 FiO_2. Conversely, high-flow systems can be used to reliably deliver low as well as high oxygen concentrations.

1. Nasal Cannula

This simple low-flow oxygen delivery device consists of two short plastic prongs arising from a hollow face piece (Figure 3.2). The prongs are inserted into the anterior nares, and oxygen is delivered into the nasopharynx. The inspired oxygen concentration is dependent on many factors, including oxygen flow rate, nasal resistance, oropharyngeal resistance, inspiratory flow rate, and tidal volume. No simple relation between nasal oxygen and inspired oxygen concentration is reliable. A high oxygen flow rate (> 6 L/min) is irritating to the nasopharynx and does not appreciably improve oxygenation. A nasal cannula is suitable for children who require only modest sup-

plemental oxygen. One disadvantage is that adequate humidification cannot be provided via the nasal cannula.

2. Nasal Catheter

A nasal catheter is a flexible, lubricated oxygen catheter with multiple holes in the distal 2 cm of the tip, which is placed into one naris and advanced posteriorly into the pharynx behind the uvula. This method of oxygen delivery is discouraged since it has no advantage over the nasal cannula, may cause hemorrhage from trauma to enlarged adenoids, and may produce gastric distention or rupture if inadvertently placed in the esophagus.

3. Oxygen Hood

An oxygen hood is a clear Plexiglas dome that encompasses the patient's head. It is well-tolerated by infants, allows easy access to the chest, trunk, and extremities, and allows control of oxygen concentration, temperature, and humidity. A gas inflow rate of $\geq$ 10–15 L/min will maintain approximately the same oxygen concentration within the hood as the gas source. As a rule, the hood is not large enough to be used with children over 1 year of age.

4. Oxygen Tent

The oxygen tent is a clear plastic shell that envelops the entire child in an increased oxygen atmosphere. It is capable of delivering in excess of .50 FiO_2 with high-flows, but there is usually difficulty in establishing a stable desired oxygen concentration because of room air entry into the tent, especially during patient manipulation. Other disadvantages include limited access to the patient and, if mist is used, difficulty in observing the patient. In practice, if an FiO_2 > .30 is needed, a tent will not be satisfactory.

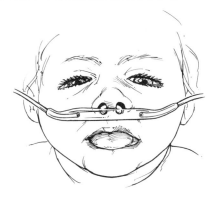

Figure 3.2. Nasal cannula.

5. Oxygen Mask

Several types of oxygen masks are used to administer a wide range of oxygen concentrations with humidification. Masks are often not tolerated by infants, but the soft vinyl pediatric mask may be accepted by children.

The simple oxygen mask is a low-flow device that will deliver from 35 to 60% oxygen with a flow rate of 6–10 L/min. The moderate oxygen concentration delivered results from the inspiratory entrainment of room air through exhalation ports in the side of the mask and between the mask and the face. The greater the inspiratory flow rate of the patient's spontaneous breaths and the lower the oxygen flow into the mask, the lower the concentration of oxygen delivered to the patient. A minimum oxygen flow of 6 L/min must be used to maintain an increased oxygen concentration and prevent rebreathing of exhaled carbon dioxide.

A *partial rebreathing* mask consists of a simple face mask with an added reservoir bag. It is useful for providing a reliable inspired oxygen concentration of 50–60%. During exhalation, fresh oxygen flows into the reservoir bag together with the first third of the patient's exhaled gases. Since this portion of the exhaled gas remains in the upper airways and does not participate in respiratory gas exchange during the prior breath, it is oxygen enriched. During inspiration the patient draws gas from the fresh oxygen inflow, from the reservoir bag, and potentially, from the room through the exhalation ports. The entrainment of room air is reduced and the rebreathing of exhaled carbon dioxide from the mask is prevented by maintaining an oxygen flow rate into the bag greater than the patient's minute ventilation (determined by a flow rate great enough to prevent the bag from completely emptying during inspiration). Generally, a flow of 10–12 L/min is required.

A *non-rebreathing mask* has 1) valves incorporated into the exhalation ports to prevent entrainment of room air during inspiration, and 2) a valve placed between the reservoir bag and mask to prevent gas flow back into the bag from the mask during exhalation. On inspiration the patient draws 100% oxygen from the reservoir and the fresh oxygen inflow. Oxygen flow into the mask is adjusted to prevent collapse of the bag. An inspired oxygen concentration of 95% can be achieved with an oxygen flow of 10–12 L/min and a well-sealed face mask.

A Venturi mask is designed to reliably and predictably provide controlled low-to-moderate (25–60%) inspired oxygen concentrations. There is little application for the use of this device in pediatric patients.

6. Face Tent

A face tent (face shield, Figure 3.3) is a high-flow soft plastic "bucket" that is often better tolerated by children than a face mask. It will deliver an oxygen concentration equal to that of the gas source if a high flow (10–15 L/min) is used. However, stable concentrations in excess of .40 FiO$_2$ are not reliable. An advantage of the face tent is that it permits access to the face (e.g., for suctioning).

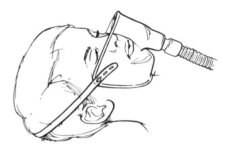

Figure 3.3. Face tent or shield.

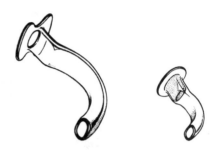

Figure 3.4. Oropharyngeal airways.

A

B

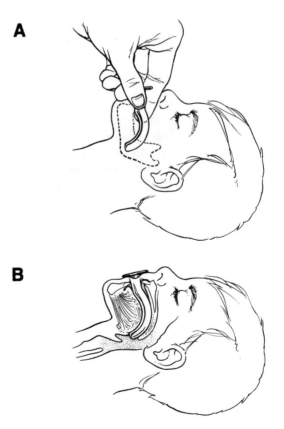

Figure 3.5. The oropharyngeal airway: Correct method of selecting the proper size. (A) Oropharyngeal airway outside; (B) Oropharyngeal airway inserted.

A

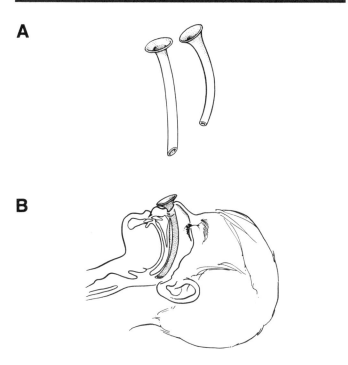

B

Figure 3.6. (A) Nasopharyngeal airways. (B) Placement of a nasopharyngeal airway.

C. Oropharyngeal Airway

An oropharyngeal airway is curved to fit over the back of the tongue to hold it away from the posterior pharyngeal wall. It may be inserted into an *unconscious* infant or child, in order to maintain airway patency, but should not be used in a conscious child since it may stimulate retching and vomiting. An oropharyngeal airway consists of a flange, a short bite block segment, and a curved body usually made of plastic and shaped to provide an air channel and suction conduit through the mouth (Figure 3.4). Sizes range from 4 to 10 cm in length (Guedel sizes 000 to 4) to fit children of all ages. The proper size for a child may be estimated by placing the oropharyngeal airway next to the face, with the flange at the level of the central incisors and the bite block segment parallel to the hard palate. The tip of the appropriate size airway should reach the angle of the jaw (Figure 3.5A and B).

The oropharyngeal airway should be inserted using a tongue depressor to hold the tongue on the floor of the mouth. If a tongue depressor is not available, the airway may be inverted for insertion into the mouth, using the posterior portion of the curved body as if it were a tongue depressor; as the airway approaches the back of the oropharynx, it is rotated into its proper position. If the oropharyngeal airway is too small or is inserted improperly, it will push the tongue posteriorly into the pharynx, obstructing the airway. If it is too large, it may obstruct the larynx. Proper head and jaw position must be maintained despite the presence of an oropharyngeal airway.

D. Nasopharyngeal Airway

A nasopharyngeal airway is a soft rubber or plastic tube that provides a conduit for air flow between the tongue and the posterior pharyngeal wall (Figure 3.6A and B). Responsive patients tolerate it better than the oropharyngeal airway. Nasopharyngeal airways are available in sizes 12 to 36 Fr.; a 12 Fr. nasopharyngeal airway (approximately the size of a 3.0 mm ET tube) will generally fit the nasopharynx of a full-term infant. The outside diameter should not be so large as to cause sustained blanching of the ala nasae. The proper length is estimated by measuring the distance from the tip of the nose to the tragus of the ear. The airway is lubricated and inserted through a nostril in a posterior direction perpendicular to the plane of the face and passed gently along the floor of the nasopharynx. Caution should be used since the airway may lacerate adenoidal tissue or the mucosa, resulting in a nose bleed that may aggravate airway obstruction and complicate airway management. Small-diameter nasopharyngeal airways may become obstructed by mucus, blood, vomitus, or the soft tissues of the pharynx, making them unreliable.

E. Suction Devices

Achieving airway patency often requires suctioning secretions, blood, vomitus, or meconium from the oropharynx, nasopharynx, or trachea. Suction may be obtained from a vacuum outlet or electrical or battery-powered portable suction device. Portable suction devices have the advantage of ease of transport but may not provide the suction power of a wall vacuum, which can exceed 300 mmHg.

Flexible plastic suction catheters are useful for the aspiration of thin secretions from an endotracheal tube, the trachea, nasopharynx, or mouth. Rigid plastic or stainless steel wide-bore suction cannulas (tonsil tips) provide more effective access to the pharynx during a crisis and are useful for the removal of thick secretions and particulate matter from the pharynx. Since vagal stimulation with resultant bradycardia may occur from catheter stimulation of the posterior pharynx, larynx, or trachea, the heart rate should be monitored during suctioning.

During endotracheal suctioning, sterile technique should be used to reduce the likelihood of airway contamination. A side opening proximally located on the suction catheter is used for on/off control of the negative pressure. The catheter should be inserted into the airway to a length just beyond the end of the endotracheal tube without negative pressure; suction is then applied by occluding the side opening while withdrawing the catheter with a rotating, twisting motion. Suction should not exceed 5 seconds and is preceded and followed by a short period of ventilation with 100% oxygen to avoid hypoxemia.

Table 3.2. Guidelines for Face Mask, Laryngoscope, and Tracheal Tube Sizes

Patient Age	Face Mask	Laryngoscope	Endotracheal Tube Size I.D. (mm)	Distance (cm): Midtrachea to Teeth	Suction Catheter (Fr)
Premature infant	0 Rendell-Baker 1 Vital Signs	Miller 0*	2.5, 3.0 Uncuffed	8	5–6
Term infant	1 Rendell Baker 2 Vital Signs	Miller 0–1* Wis-Hipple 1 Robertshaw 0	3.0, 3.5 Uncuffed	10	6–8
6 months			3.5, 4.0 Uncuffed	12	8
1 year	2 Rendell-Baker	Wis-Hipple 1–1/2 Robertshaw 1	4.0, 4.5 Uncuffed	12	8
2 years	3 Vital Signs	Miller 2 Flagg 2	4.5 Uncuffed	14	8
4 years	3 Rendell-Baker		5.0 Uncuffed	16	10
6 years	4 Vital Signs		5.5 Uncuffed	16	10
8 years	Small Trimar	Miller 2 MacIntosh 2	6.0 Cuffed or Uncuffed	18	10
10 years			6.5 Cuffed or Uncuffed	18	12
12 years	Ohio 2 or 3 5 Vital Signs	MacIntosh 3	7.0 Cuffed	20	12
Adolescent	Ohio 3 or 4	MacIntosh 3 Miller 3	7.0, 8.0 Cuffed	22	12

*Oxyscope modifications are available for Miller 0 and 1 blades. They may reduce the likelihood of hypoxemia during laryngoscopy in infants.

III. Airway Adjuncts for the Patient in Respiratory Failure or Arrest

A. General Principles

The infant or child with absent ventilation should be easy to recognize and requires prompt resuscitative measures. Early recognition of *inadequate* ventilation is assessed by careful auscultation and by evaluation of the **level of consciousness, work of breathing, respiratory rate,** and mucus membrane **color.** Recognition of sweating, grunting, or nasal flaring (see Chapter 1) is also essential. If respiratory failure is imminent, supportive measures must be instituted. The basic approach is the same as in BLS: 1) Open the **A**IRWAY; 2) begin **B**REATHING using an appropriate adjunct that will deliver the highest available oxygen concentration and adequate ventilation; then 3) assess the **C**IRCULATION.

Impending respiratory failure is not always readily apparent from a single examination. Rather, it is best identified when the physical examination and laboratory data (e.g., arterial blood gases) at a given time are interpreted in the context of previous examinations and data and the patient's history. When a trend is appreciated, specific intervention will frequently prevent respiratory failure. However, when overt respiratory failure, as defined clinically or by blood gases, occurs, there is only one therapeutic modality: assisted ventilation. It should be implemented without delay.

B. Ventilation Masks and Cricoid Pressure

A ventilation face mask enables a rescuer to ventilate and oxygenate a patient with a ventilating device. It can be used with an oropharyngeal or nasopharyngeal airway during spontaneous, assisted, or controlled ventilation.

A mask consists of a rubber or plastic body, a standardized 15/22 mm connecting port, and a rim or face seal. A mask used for older children and adults has a soft, inflatable cuff with a relatively large under-mask volume. In infants and small children, the mask should have a small under-mask volume to decrease dead space and prevent rebreathing of exhaled gases. Ideally, the mask should be transparent, permitting the rescuer to observe the color of the child's lips and to recognize regurgitation quickly.

Face masks are available in a variety of sizes (Table 3.2). The proper mask size is selected to provide an air-tight seal on the face; the mask should extend from the bridge of the nose to the cleft of the chin, enveloping the nose and mouth but avoiding compression of the eyes (Figure 3.7). Failure to obtain a tight mask fit results in a lowered inspired oxygen concentration during spontaneous respiration and precludes efficient assisted or controlled ventilation. The mask is held on the face with a one-handed head-tilt/chin-lift maneuver (Figure 3.8). In infants and toddlers, the jaw is supported with the base of the third finger; caution is used to avoid compression in the submental triangle, which can result in airway obstruction. In older children, the fingertips of the third, fourth, and fifth fingers are placed on the ridge of the mandible to hold the jaw forward and extend the head (one-handed jaw-thrust maneuver). A two-person procedure with one person holding the mask to the face and the second person ventilating (Figure 3.9) may be more effective in maintaining a tight mask fit.[10]

During mask ventilation, the degree of extension of the head required to open the airway varies. Infants and toddlers are best maintained in a neutral sniffing position without hyperextension of the head. The rescuer may have to move the head gently through a range of extension to find the optimal position. Hyperextension is avoided since it can produce airway obstruction.

During assisted or controlled ventilation applied through a ventilating face mask or by mouth-to-mouth (or mouth-to-nose) rescue breathing, inflation of the stomach occurs frequently, particularly when high airway pressures are generated within the pharynx. This is likely when assisted or controlled ventilation is provided in the presence of partial airway obstruction or when an excessive inspiratory flow rate or ventilation pressure is used. Gastric distention should be avoided since it predisposes to regurgitation and aspiration of stomach contents and may prevent adequate ventilation by limiting downward displacement of the diaphragm.

Gastric inflation can be minimized by the application of *cricoid pressure* (Sellick maneuver) during assisted or controlled ventilation (Figure 3.10).[11,12] This maneuver occludes the proximal esophagus by application of pressure to the cricoid cartilage, pushing it posteriorly and,

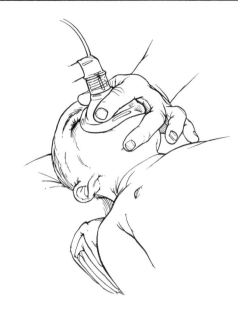

Figure 3.8. One-handed face mask application technique.

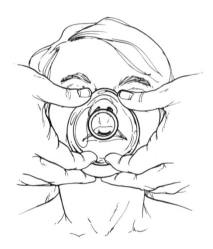

Figure 3.9. Two-handed face mask application technique. A second person is needed to ventilate.

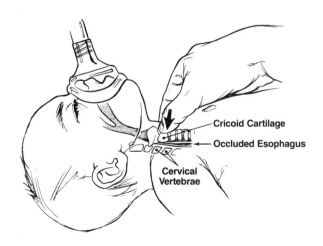

Cricoid Cartilage

Occluded Esophagus

Cervical Vertebrae

Figure 3.10. Cricoid pressure (Sellick maneuver) with mask.

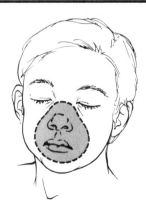

Figure 3.7. Area of the face for a face mask.

thus, compressing the esophagus between the cricoid ring and the cervical spine. The cricoid cartilage is the first tracheal ring and is located by palpating a prominent horizontal band inferior to the thyroid cartilage and cricothyroid membrane. Cricoid pressure is applied by a second rescuer to unconscious infants and children using one fingertip in infants and the thumb and index finger in children. Excessive pressure must be avoided because it may produce tracheal compression and obstruction in infants. Cricoid pressure is released once endotracheal intubation is accomplished.

C. Endotracheal Airway

When prolonged ventilation is required, or when adequate ventilation cannot otherwise be achieved, the face mask is replaced by an endotracheal tube, which has the following advantages: 1) It isolates the larynx and trachea from the pharynx, preventing gastric distension and minimizing the risk of aspiration; 2) it permits suctioning of airway secretions, blood, mucus, or meconium; 3) it provides a means of administering several resuscitation medications (see Chapter 5), and 4) it permits application of positive end-expiratory pressure (PEEP). PEEP is used to improve ventilation–perfusion matching and to increase the functional residual capacity of the lungs; it is most often used in conditions where increased FiO_2 does not improve oxygenation.[13]

1. The Endotracheal Tube

The endotracheal tube should be sterile, disposable, and constructed of translucent polyvinyl chloride (Figure 3.11). An endotracheal tube of uniform internal diameter is preferred to one that is tapered; the Cole shouldered tracheal tube is not recommended since it may cause laryngeal injury when used for extended periods because the proximal portion of the tube places excessive pressure on the trachea at the level of the cricoid. A standard 15-mm adaptor is firmly affixed to the proximal end for attachment to a ventilating device. The distal end may include an opening in the side wall (Murphy eye) to reduce the likelihood of complete tube obstruction if the end opening is blocked. The tube should have distance (cm) markings along its length for use as reference points to aid in placement and to detect accidental tube movement. In some tubes a vocal cord marker is placed at the level of the glottic opening to ensure that the tip of the tube is in a midtracheal position.

A cuffed endotracheal tube should have a low-pressure, high-volume cuff and is generally indicated only in older children (> 8 years). In children less than 8 years, the circular narrowing at the level of the cricoid cartilage serves as a functional cuff. The cuff should be inflated to the point at which an audible air leak at the larynx just disappears. A properly selected uncuffed endotracheal tube will allow a minimal air leak at the cricoid ring; the absence of an air leak indicates that excessive pressure is likely to occur at the cricoid cartilage.

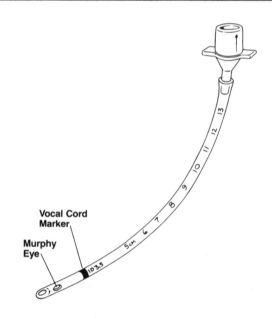

Figure 3.11. Endotracheal tube with distance markers.

Several methods and formulas have been developed for estimating the correct tube size. In one such formula (used for children > 1 year) tube size (internal diameter in millimeters) may be approximated as follows:[14]

$$I.D. = \frac{16 + \text{Patient's age in years}}{4}$$

In an alternate formula, 18 is substituted for 16. A 3.0-mm- or 3.5-mm-I.D. tube is used in term newborns and small infants; a 4.0-mm-I.D. tube in the first year of life. A simple visual estimation of appropriate tube size can be made by choosing an endotracheal tube with an outside diameter approximating the diameter of the child's little finger. These are only estimates; therefore, tubes 0.5-mm smaller and larger than the estimated tube size should be readily available. Recommended tube sizes are given in Table 3.2.

2. The Laryngoscope

The laryngoscope consists of a handle with a battery and a blade with a light source used to expose the glottis by moving the tongue laterally and compressing its base into the floor of the mouth. Adult and pediatric laryngoscope handles fit all blades interchangeably and differ only in handle diameter. The blade may be curved or straight (Figure 3.12); several sizes are available (Table 3.2). A straight blade is preferred for infants since it provides greater displacement of the tongue into the floor of the mouth and better visualization of the relatively cephalad and anterior glottis. A curved blade is preferred for the older child since its broader base and flange facilitate displacement of the tongue.

3. Intubation Technique

Laryngoscopy permits a visual axis through the mouth and pharynx to the larynx through which an endotracheal

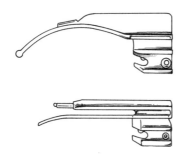

Figure 3.12. Laryngoscope blades — curved and straight.

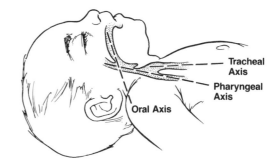

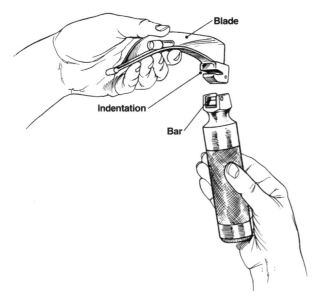

Figure 3.13. Attaching a blade to a laryngoscope handle. The blade locks into place when it is properly engaged.

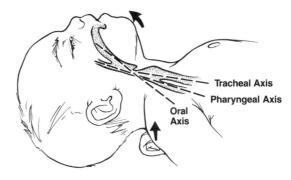

Figure 3.14. Alignment of the mouth, pharynx, and trachea for intubation.

tube, suction catheter, or Magill forceps can be passed for tracheal intubation, suctioning, or extraction of foreign material. Ventilation with a bag–valve–mask device using 100% oxygen should always precede an attempt to intubate. Since ventilation is interrupted during intubation, attempts to intubate should not exceed 30 seconds and heart rate should be monitored during the procedure. Longer attempts may produce profound hypoxemia, especially in infants, whose small lung volumes and high rates of oxygen use rapidly consume oxygen reserves.

Prior to laryngoscopy, the laryngoscope and suction equipment should be checked to ensure that they are in working order. A selection of blades should be available and the proper size blade selected (Table 3.2). The blade is attached to the handle by inserting the U-shaped indentation of the blade onto the small bar at the end of the handle (Figure 3.13). After the indentation is aligned with the bar, the blade is pressed forward to clip it onto the bar. The blade is then elevated until it snaps into position perpendicular to the handle, at which time the light on the flange of the blade should go on. If it is dim,

flickers, or does not light, the blade may be improperly seated on the handle or the fault may lie with the bulb or the batteries (contained in the handle). Fiberoptic technology is available for laryngoscopic illumination.

A malleable, yet rigid stylet may be inserted into the tracheal tube to shape it to a desired configuration. To avoid airway trauma during intubation, the tip of the stylet *must not* extend beyond the distal end of the tracheal tube. The stylet may be lubricated for ease of withdrawal once the endotracheal tube is positioned.

Heart rate should be continuously monitored during intubation since mechanical stimulation of the airway may induce reflex bradyarrhythmias in the infant and young child. If bradycardia occurs (heart rate < 80 beats/min in the infant and < 60 beats/min in the child), the procedure should be interrupted and the patient ventilated with 100% oxygen by face mask. The incidence of bradyarrhythmias during intubation may be reduced by pretreatment with intravenous atropine (0.02 mg/kg). However, bradycardia is an early sign of hypoxemia, and atropine will blunt this early warning detector. Atropine is recommended for intubating the spontaneously breathing infant or child; time does not permit its use for the apneic child.

To achieve direct visualization of the glottis, the axes of the mouth, pharynx, and trachea must be aligned (Figure 3.14). This is accomplished by flexion of the neck on the shoulders and simultaneous extension of the head on the

A

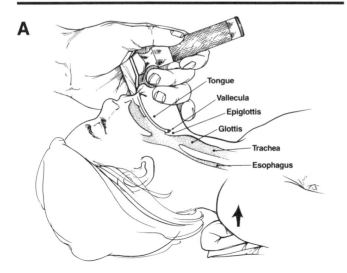

Tongue
Vallecula
Epiglottis
Glottis
Trachea
Esophagus

B

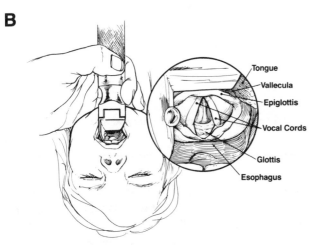

Tongue
Vallecula
Epiglottis
Vocal Cords
Glottis
Esophagus

Figure 3.15. (A) Introduction of laryngoscope with anatomic landmarks. (B) Operator's view of the internal anatomy.

neck, i.e., the "sniffing position," unless there is a suspicion of head or neck injury, in which case the neutral position must be maintained using manual in-line cervical stabilization. The laryngoscope handle is held in the left hand, and the blade is inserted into the mouth, following the natural contour of the pharynx along the right side of the tongue (Figure 3.15A and B). Once the tip of the blade is at the back of the tongue, control of the tongue is achieved by moving the blade from the right side of the mouth to the middle. This left lateral movement provides a channel in the right one-third of the mouth, through which the endotracheal tube will be passed (Figure 3.15B). When a curved blade is used, its tip is placed in the vallecula above the epiglottis (Figure 3.16A). When a straight blade is used, its tip is passed below the epiglottis to rest above the glottic opening (Figure 3.16B). Once properly positioned, blade traction is exerted upward in the direction of the long axis of the handle to displace the base of the tongue and the epiglottis anteriorly, exposing the glottis. The handle must not be used with a prying or

levering motion, nor should the upper gums or teeth be used as a fulcrum.

The tracheal tube is inserted from the right corner of the mouth to avoid visual obstruction of the glottic opening by the tube. In this way, the rescuer should see insertion of the tube through the glottic opening. The glottic marker (if present) is placed at the level of the vocal cords, which places the tube in the mid-tracheal position. Endotracheal tube position must be confirmed by a chest x-ray. Cuffed endotracheal tubes are inserted until the cuff is located just below the vocal cords.

Proper positioning of the tube must be confirmed immediately by 1) observing symmetrical chest movements, 2) auscultating equal breath sounds over each lateral chest wall, 3) noting the absence of breath sounds over the stomach, and 4) observing condensation in the endotracheal tube during exhalation. If these criteria are not met and/or epigastric distension occurs with ventilation, esophageal intubation is suspected and the tube should be removed. Ventilation should be maintained by bag–valve–mask. If chest movement or breath sounds are asymmetrical (particularly if audible only over the right lung), bronchial intubation is suspected and the tube should be slowly withdrawn until bilateral breath sounds are present; withdrawing 1–2 cm further should then place the tube close to the midtracheal position.

If the tube is properly placed but inadequate lung expansion occurs or inadequate ventilation is documented on an arterial blood gas, a search for one of the following should be initiated:

1. The tube is too small and a large air leak is present at the glottic opening. This should be obvious from auscultation over the neck. If a large leak is present, the tube should be replaced with a larger tube; in the child over 8 years, the cuff of the endotracheal tube should be inflated until the air leak just disappears.
2. The pop-off valve on the resuscitation bag is not depressed and ventilation is escaping into the atmosphere. This is a problem particularly in the victim with poorly compliant lungs, such as the near-drowning victim or the child with pulmonary edema.[15]
3. There is a leak in the bag–valve device. This may occur at any one of a number of connections in the device and should be carefully evaluated. Disconnecting the bag–valve device and occluding the endotracheal connection while compressing the bag will reveal the presence of a leak.
4. The operator is giving too shallow a breath; this is easily assessed by giving a larger breath.

Following intubation, the tube should be secured to the patient's face with benzoin and tape to prevent accidental extubation. Before beginning to tape the tube in place, correct position should be reconfirmed by auscultation and the distance marker noted at the lips to avoid accidental displacement of the tube during taping. (See Table 3.2 for distance from mid-trachea to teeth.) As soon as convenient, a chest x-ray should be obtained to confirm proper tube placement.

Orotracheal intubation is preferred during resuscitation because it can be performed rapidly. While technically more difficult, nasotracheal intubation should be considered following successful resuscitation if extended ventilatory support is likely. A description of the technique can be found elsewhere.[16]

D. Esophageal Obturator Airway

Esophageal obturator airways (EOA) are not recommended for the pediatric patient because of the variability in esophageal lengths and face mask sizes required for this age group.

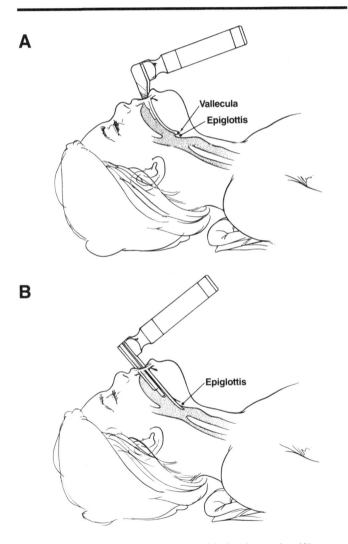

Figure 3.16. Position of laryngoscope blade when using (A) a curved blade vs. (B) a straight blade.

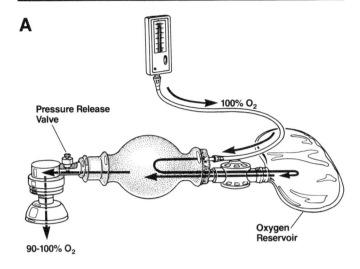

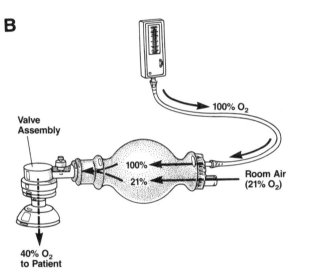

Figure 3.17. Self-inflating bag–valve (A) with and (B) without an oxygen reservoir.

E. Self-Inflating Bag–Valve Ventilation Devices

A bag–valve device with a face mask provides a rapid means of ventilating the patient; ventilation can be achieved in an emergency even in the absence of a source of oxygen.

The self-inflating bag–valve ventilation device[9] consists of two valves (Figure 3.17) and a self-inflating bag and may be used in conjunction with a mask or endotracheal tube. Such devices are available in sizes for infants, children, and adults. The recoil allows the self-inflating bag to refill independent of inflow from a gas source. During reinflation, a gas intake valve opens, entraining room air, or supplemental oxygen if a fresh oxygen inflow reservoir is provided. During bag compression, the gas intake valve closes and a second valve opens to permit gas flow to the patient. During patient exhalation the bag outlet valve (non-rebreathing valve) closes and the patient's exhaled gases are vented into the atmosphere, thus avoiding rebreathing and carbon dioxide retention. An inability to ventilate or a rebreathing of CO_2 may occur if secretions or vomitus interfere with proper functioning of the non-rebreathing valve.

A bag–valve device delivers room air (21% oxygen) unless supplemental oxygen is provided. Pediatric bag–valve devices without oxygen reservoirs deliver 30–80% oxygen at a 10 L/min oxygen inflow.[17] To deliver a consistently higher oxygen concentration, a bag–valve device should be equipped with an oxygen reservoir. Oxygen concentrations from 60 to 95% can be provided by reservoir-equipped bag–valve devices; 10–15 L/min of oxygen flow are required to maintain an adequate oxygen volume in the reservoir and should be considered the minimal flow rate.[17] Adult bag–valve devices, which have larger reinflating bags, require an oxygen inflow of 15 L/min or greater to reliably deliver high oxygen concentrations. High oxygen flow rates, however, may cause some spring-loaded ball or disk outlet valves to chatter or stick. If this occurs, the flow rate should be reduced to the maximum rate that does not cause chattering or sticking.

Many bags are equipped with a pressure-limited pop-off valve set at 35–45 cmH$_2$O in an effort to avoid barotrauma. Those used for resuscitation should have no pop-off valve or one that is easily occluded since pressures required for ventilation during CPR may exceed the pop-off limit.[15] In the patient with poorly compliant (stiff) lungs, delivered tidal volume may be insufficient, as assessed by an absence of adequate chest rise when the pop-off valve is not occluded.[17] Pop-off valves may be occluded by depressing the valve with a finger during ventilation or, in some devices, twisting the valve into a closed position. Ventilation pressure can best be monitored by having a manometer in line with the bag–valve device.

Selecting an appropriately sized bag–valve device is necessary so that the device conveys to the operator a sense of the patient's lung compliance. Sudden decreases in lung compliance may indicate 1) right mainstem intubation, 2) an obstructed tube, or 3) pneumothorax. When using assisted ventilation, tidal volume should be 10–15 mL/kg. Therefore, a bag volume of 250–750 mL should be used since larger bags make it difficult to regulate the small tidal volumes.

Bag–valve devices with a fish-mouth or leaf-flap operated outlet (non-rebreathing) valve cannot be used reliably to provide supplemental oxygen during spontaneous ventilation. Although these valves can open during inspiration, allowing the child to inspire the gas mixture contained in the bag, many children cannot sustain the increased work of breathing required to open the outlet valve. Bag–valve devices with spring-loaded disk or ball-operated outlet valves will *not* open during patient inspiration; gas is delivered only when the bag is compressed. Thus, self-inflating bag–valve devices are *not* useful as sources of supplemental oxygen for the spontaneously breathing infant or child.

Positive end-expiratory pressure (PEEP) may be provided during controlled or assisted ventilation by the addition of a compatible spring-loaded ball or disk or a magnetic disk PEEP valve to the bag–valve outlet. Bag–valve devices equipped with PEEP valves are *not* to be used to provide continuous positive airway pressure (CPAP) in the spontaneously breathing child since excessive negative inspiratory pressure would be required to open the outlet valve.

F. Anesthesia Ventilation Systems

Anesthesia ventilating systems[18] consist of a reservoir bag, an overflow port, corrugated tubing, a fresh gas inflow port, and a standard 15/22-mm connector for mask or tracheal tube connection (Figure 3.18). The overflow port usually includes an adjustable clamp or valve. The reservoir bag volume for infants is 500 mL; for children, 1,000–1,500 mL; for adults, 1,500–2,000 mL.

These ventilation devices require more experience to use than the self-inflating bag since the fresh gas flow and outlet valve must be carefully adjusted. The composition of inspired gas depends on fresh gas flow since a non-rebreathing valve is absent. A high flow is required to flush exhaled gases through the corrugated tubing to the flow control valve and reservoir bag. The flow control valve must be adjusted to maintain volume in the reservoir bag yet permit a high oxygen inflow rate to wash out exhaled gases. Failure to open the flow control valve may result in high airway pressure and, thus, pulmonary barotrauma, or insufficient washout of exhaled gases, which result in rebreathing and hypercapnia. The oxygen inflow must not be adjusted to an insufficient flow rate to compensate for a flow control valve that is too tightly closed. Similarly, it is improper to close the flow control valve in an effort to compensate for an insufficient O_2 inflow rate. In both instances, rebreathing of exhaled gases may occur. To avoid barotrauma, an in-line pressure manometer should be used. Opening the valve too far allows the reservoir to collapse and prevents ventilation of the patient until it refills. For these reasons, the anesthesia bag should be used only by individuals with proper training and experience.

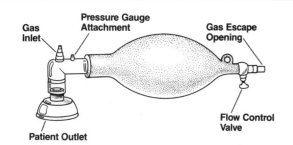

Figure 3.18. Anesthesia ventilation bag. (A) Patient outlet, (B) gas escape opening, (C) gas inlet, (D) pressure gauge attachment, (E) flow control valve.

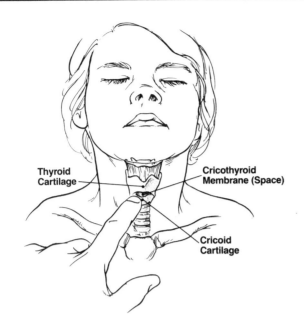

Figure 3.19. Cricothyroid membrane anatomy.

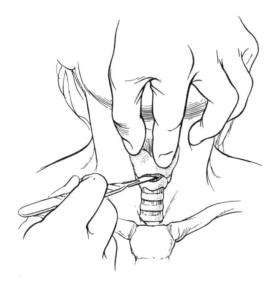

Figure 3.20. Surgical cricothyrotomy.

Fresh gas flow should be at least 2 L/min in patients < 10 kg, 4.0 L/min in patients 10–50 kg, and 6 L/min in patients above 50 kg. Increasing fresh gas flow decreases rebreathing of carbon dioxide and is an effective means of preventing hypercarbia without increasing tidal volume or respiratory rate.

Anesthesia ventilating systems can be used to provide supplemental oxygen during spontaneous respiration, even in small infants, since there are no flow valves for the infant to open. When used as sources of supplemental oxygen in spontaneously breathing patients, however, they are less efficient in removing exhaled carbon dioxide; and fresh gas flow rates should be at least three times the patient's minute ventilation. PEEP or CPAP may also

be provided by partial closure of the adjustable overflow valve until the desired level of end-expiratory pressure is achieved.

G. Oxygen-Powered Breathing Devices

Oxygen-powered breathing devices are *not* recommended for pediatric use because tidal volume is difficult to control and high airway pressures may develop, producing gastric distention (with mask ventilation) or tension pneumothorax.

H. Cricothyrotomy

Cricothyrotomy is a technique that is infrequently required to provide an open airway and ventilation in children with upper airway obstruction due to a foreign body, severe orofacial injuries, or laryngeal fracture. Other airway opening methods, including the repositioning of the head and jaw, the use of an oropharyngeal airway, and tracheal intubation, when properly performed, will permit ventilation under most circumstances. While the place of cricothyrotomy in pediatric airway management should be limited, the technique is presented for those highly skilled medical providers in hospital settings who encounter cases of complete upper airway obstruction that cannot be treated with other techniques.

Cricothyrotomy may be effective in older children and adults because the site of obstruction in these groups is most frequently at or above the glottis. In children less than approximately 8 years of age, the subglottic cricoid ring, inferior to the cricothyroid membrane, forms the narrowest segment of the airway; and cricothyrotomy may therefore not be effective. However, since a rescuer cannot predict the exact site of foreign-body or traumatic obstruction, cricothyrotomy should not be withheld when other methods have failed to provide airway patency.

The cricothyroid membrane extends from the cricoid to the thyroid cartilage (Figure 3.19). It is located by palpating for an anterior and midline transverse indentation between the two cartilages. The relatively avascular membrane can be punctured and the underlying trachea entered percutaneously, using a large-bore cannula. The cannula is directed in the midline caudally and posteriorly at a 45-degree angle. Aspiration of air signifies entry into the trachea. The cannula is advanced into the trachea and connected to an appropriate ventilating device. Cricothyrotomy may also be accomplished surgically with a short, horizontal incision (Figure 3.20) made over the cricothyroid membrane, which is then spread apart. A small-bore cannula (e.g., 3.0-mm endotracheal tube) is inserted into the tracheal opening.

If effective ventilation and oxygenation are to be achieved through a cricothyrotomy, the insertion of a transtracheal cannula of adequate size and the use of an appropriate ventilating device are mandatory. Ventilation and oxygenation with a bag–valve device can be achieved in children and small adults provided a 3.0-mm-I.D. or larger transtracheal cannula is used.[19] Large-bore intravenous catheters, 14 or 16 gauge, have been used to accomplish percutaneous cricothyrotomy in adults. The high resistance to air flow offered by these small diameter catheters prohibits effective ventilation by a bag–valve device coupled to the intravenous catheter with a 15-mm endotracheal tube connector. Ventilation and oxygenation via 14- or 16-gauge intravenous catheters require the use of specialized high-flow jet oxygen ventilation devices. These specialized ventilation devices are not available to most rescuers. Moreover, published experience with percutaneous catheter cricothyrotomy in infants and small children is lacking and recommendations for the selection of appropriate size intravenous catheters for this purpose in children are not available. For these reasons, the use of intravenous catheters to achieve percutaneous cricothyrotomy is not generally recommended. This technique will be of use only to physicians who are trained in pediatric invasive techniques and who have access to jet ventilation devices.[20–27]

IV. Airway Emergencies in the Patient With an Artificial Airway

A. Assessment

As previously discussed, airway management is crucial to the prevention of cardiac arrest and successful resuscitation of the patient with respiratory failure. The airway must be opened and ventilation assisted or controlled. *Frequent reassessment* of adequacy of ventilation and oxygenation is essential and includes:

1. observation of symmetrical chest wall expansion;
2. auscultation of equal bilateral breath sounds;
3. improvement of patient color and perfusion; and
4. objective measurement of the efficacy of ventilation by obtaining a blood gas.

B. Managing Airway Emergencies

Patients with an artificial airway (endotracheal or tracheostomy tube) are at particular risk for a variety of problems that may result in life-threatening loss of airway function. These problems include 1) loss of gas supply to the tube, 2) occlusion or kinking of the tube, and 3) displacement of the tube (either too far down or out of the trachea). Precautions must be taken to reduce the probability of such events, and patients must be monitored carefully so that events are detected early and appropriate action can be taken to prevent a problem from becoming an emergency.

When a problem is detected, the first priority is a rapid assessment of the patient's status. Adequacy of air exchange and oxygenation are evaluated by observing the patient and the monitoring devices (i.e., pulse oximeter or transcutaneous oxygen electrode) and by auscultating the chest for bilaterally equal and adequate breath sounds and for the heart rate. This information will determine the rapidity of the response that is required.

The second priority is to determine the probable cause of the problem. Tube position is evaluated by visual inspection and auscultation. Any gas delivery system (e.g., ventilator) in use should be temporarily disconnected and the patient *ventilated manually* with a resuscitation bag, using 100% oxygen. Auscultation during manual ventilation will help to assess tube patency and position (an endotracheal tube may be too far down the airway, with obstruction of the left main bronchus). If breath sounds are poor and there is no movement of the chest with manual inflation, the tube has been displaced from the trachea or is obstructed (in which case there will be high resistance to manual inflation). If the tube is obstructed, an attempt should be made to suction the tube, using a relatively large catheter and making certain that the suction catheter will pass beyond the end of the tube. After suctioning, a repeat manual ventilation and assessments of breath sounds, airway resistance, and adequacy of chest movement are performed. If the patient has a tracheostomy tube with an inner cannula, the cannula should be removed; this may relieve the obstruction. If the tube appears to be properly positioned and adequate ventilation is obtained by manual inflation, it may be assumed that the problem is in the gas delivery system. The patient should be manually ventilated until the problem can be identified and corrected.

If the tube is occluded and ventilation cannot be established by suctioning, then the tube *must* be removed and replaced. The patient is ventilated by bag and mask until preparations for reintubation are complete. Likewise, if the tube is displaced out of the trachea, the patient is manually ventilated with bag and mask and then reintubated. Reintubation should be done deliberately and carefully; it should be a semi-elective procedure except for the rare situation when ventilation cannot be achieved in any other way.

Patients with tracheostomy tubes often present medical

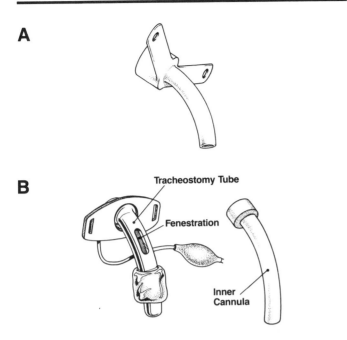

A

B

Tracheostomy Tube

Fenestration

Inner
Cannula

Figure 3.21. Tracheostomy tubes — (A) plastic and (B) metal with inner cannula.

personnel with more problems than those intubated with oral or nasal tubes, although this is due primarily to lack of experience with tracheostomy tubes rather than an inherent problem with tracheostomies. Once the principles are understood, it should be easier to deal with a tracheostomy tube than with any other endotracheal tube.

Tracheostomy tubes (Figure 3.21) may be either plastic or metal. The metal tubes have much thinner walls than the plastic and do not have a built-in 15-mm endotracheal tube connector. All metal tubes have an inner cannula, which can be easily removed for cleaning or if the tube becomes obstructed. Plastic tubes used in pediatric patients usually do not have inner cannulas, and if these tubes become occluded, they must be removed and replaced with a clean tube. The plastic tubes usually are equipped with a 15-mm connector so that they may be easily connected to an oxygen delivery system.

Suctioning a tracheostomy tube is simpler than suctioning an endotracheal tube since the former is much shorter. It should not require more than 3 or 4 seconds to suction a tracheostomy tube. As with endotracheal tubes, irrigation of the tube with a small amount of sterile saline may be helpful if secretions are very thick.

Tracheostomy tubes are held in position by ties (usually made of twill tape) extending from either side of the tube and tied around the neck. The ties must be removed or cut before the tube can be removed from the trachea. Patients with tracheostomy tubes should have a pair of scissors (and a clean tube prepared with ties) handy at all times for emergency use. The patient should be positioned with the neck somewhat extended to facilitate

access to the tracheostomy tube. Once the ties are cut, the tube may be removed from the trachea by simply grasping the tube and guiding it out.

Prior to reinserting a clean tracheostomy tube, the stoma and trachea should be suctioned with a catheter. This is especially helpful in emergency situations since thick secretions may have accumulated in the trachea around the tube and may be pushed back down the trachea by the new tube (thus occluding it). The stoma may be held open, if necessary, by gentle downward and lateral traction from two fingers placed below and to either side of the stoma. If the patient is not breathing spontaneously, bag and mask ventilation must be provided until preparations for recannulation are complete. (It may be necessary to place a finger over the stoma to prevent air escape.) If there is total upper airway obstruction and the tracheostomy stoma is the only functioning airway, mouth-to-stoma ventilation may be necessary.

The new tracheostomy tube is placed into the stoma and gently guided into position in the trachea. Usually the tube passes easily if the stoma is well healed. Because of the hazard of inadvertently pushing the tube into a paratracheal location, metal tubes should contain an obturator before attempting to insert the tube into the trachea. Plastic tubes have a much thicker wall, and obturators are rarely needed. During passage of the tube into the trachea, it is helpful to be able to hear air movement through the tube (this is lost if an obturator is used). Once the tube is in position, its patency is rapidly assessed, the patient is ventilated manually, and the ties are secured to keep the tube in the trachea. The ties should be tied snug against the neck so that a finger can be slipped under the tie but not so tightly that venous return is obstructed.

Sometimes when a tube is being replaced, difficulty is encountered in passing the tube through the stoma. There are several appropriate responses to this. The simplest and perhaps best approach is to pass a suction catheter through the new tracheostomy tube and then insert the end of the catheter through the stoma into the trachea. The small size of the catheter should make this very easy, and suctioning will help to ensure placement of the catheter in the trachea. The tracheostomy tube is then passed into the trachea, using the catheter as a guide. If a catheter is present to guide the tube, then much more pressure can be used to insert the tube through a tight stoma. Lubrication of the stoma with a mixture of sterile water and soluble lubricant also helps.

Alternative methods for recannulation include the use of a smaller size tracheostomy tube (with later replacement of the appropriate size) and the use of endotracheal tubes. The advantages of using an endotracheal tube in an emergency situation are the wide range of sizes available and the fact that the tips of endotracheal tubes are beveled, thus facilitating entry through a tight stoma. Additionally, condensation of expired air in the tube will provide visual reassurance of the continuity of the lumen of the tube with that of the trachea.

If recannulation cannot be accomplished despite these measures, then the patient should be *intubated orally* with an endotracheal tube. The tracheostomy tube can be reinserted later under controlled conditions. Another technique that may be useful in very difficult situations is that of passing a flexible bronchoscope of appropriate size through the tracheostomy tube, then through the stoma, and using the bronchoscope as a guide to pass the tube into the trachea.

In patients whose tracheostomy stoma has not yet healed (usually the first week after tracheostomy), there may be much more difficulty in recannulation after accidental or deliberate decannulation. In this circumstance, it is not uncommon for the tube to be placed into the paratracheal tissues rather than the trachea. Ventilation into the paratracheal space is likely to result in a tension pneumothorax. Most surgeons place temporary traction sutures at the lateral margins of the tracheal incision — which may be used to assist in recannulation. If such sutures are present, then gentle traction laterally will help to open the stoma and facilitate recannulation. Vigorous traction may break the sutures or damage the trachea. In general, it is wise to use a suction catheter to guide the new tube into place since it is much less likely that a catheter will create a false tract. If one or two attempts to replace the tube fail, the patient should be *intubated orally* and the tracheostomy tube replaced by the surgeon or someone especially skilled in airway management.

References

1. Lewis JK, Minter MG, Eshelman SJ, Witte MK: Outcome of pediatric resuscitation. *Ann Emerg Med* 12:297, 1983.
2. Eisenberg M, Bergner L, Hallstrom A: Epidemiology of cardiac arrest and resuscitation in children. *Ann Emerg Med* 12:672,1983.
3. Ludwig S, Kettrick RG, Parker M: Pediatric cardiopulmonary resuscitation. A Review of 130 cases. *Clin Pediatr* 23:71, 1984.
4. Wark H, Overton JH: A paediatric "cardiac arrest" survey. *Br J Anaesth* 56:1271, 1984.
5. Torphy DE, Minter MG, Thompson BM: Cardiorespiratory arrest and resuscitation of children. *Am J Dis Child* 138:1099, 1984.
6. O'Rourke PP: Outcome of children who are apneic and pulseless in the emergency room. *Crit Care Med* 14:466, 1986.
7. Eckenhoff JE: Some anatomic considerations of the infant larynx influencing endotracheal anesthesia. *Anesthesiology* 12:401, 1951.
8. Davis HW, Gartner JC, Galvis AG, et al: Acute upper airway obstruction: Croup and epiglottitis. *Pediatr Clin N Am* 28:859, 1981.
9. McPherson SP: *Respiratory Therapy Equipment*, ed 3. St. Louis, CV Mosby Co, 1985, pp 74–112, 178–204.
10. Jesudian MC, Harrison RR, Keenan RL, et al: Bag–valve–mask ventilation: Two rescuers are better than one: Preliminary report. *Crit Care Med* 13:122, 1985.
11. Sellick BA: Cricoid pressure to control regurgitation of stomach contents during induction of anaesthesia. *Lancet* 2:404, 1961.
12. Salem MR, Wong AY, Mani M, Sellick BA: Efficacy of cricoid pressure in preventing gastric inflation during bag–mask ventilation in paediatric patients. *Anesthesiology* 40:96, 1974.
13. Tyler DC: Positive end-expiratory pressure: A review. *Crit Care Med* 11:300, 1983.
14. Lee KW, Templeton JJ, Dougas R: Tracheal tube size and postoperative croup in children. *Anesthesiology* 53:S325, 1980.
15. Hirschman AM, Kravath RE: Venting vs. ventilating: A danger of manual resuscitation bags. *Chest* 82:369, 1982.
16. Endotracheal intubation, in Smith RM (ed): *Anesthesia for Infants and Children*. St. Louis, CV Mosby Co, 1980; p 164.
17. Finer NN, Barrington KJ, Al-Fadley F, Peters KL: Limitations of self-inflating resuscitators. *Pediatrics* 77:417, 1986.
18. Dorsch JA, Dorsch SE: *Understanding Anesthesia Equipment*, ed 2, Baltimore, Williams and Wilkins, 1984, pp 182–196.
19. Neff CC, Pfister RC, Van Sonnenberg E: Percutaneous transtracheal ventilation: Experimental and practical aspects. *J Trauma* 23:84–90, 1983.
20. Levinson MM, Scuderi PE, Gibson RL, Comer PB: Emergency percutaneous transtracheal ventilation (PTV). *JACEP* 8:396, 1979.
21. Spoerel WE, Narayanan PS, Singh NP: Transtracheal ventilation. *Br J Anaesth* 43:932, 1971.
22. Jacobs HB: Emergency percutaneous transtracheal catheter and ventilator. *J Trauma* 12:50, 1972.
23. Smith RB: Transtracheal ventilation during anesthesia. *Anesth Analg* 53:225, 1974.
24. Smith RB, Myers EN, Sherman H: Transtracheal ventilation in pediatric patients; case reports. *Br J Anaesth* 46:313, 1974.
25. Miyasaka K, Sloan IA, Froese AB: An evaluation of the jet injector (Sanders) technique for bronchoscopy in pediatric patients. *Can Anaesth Soc J* 27:117, 1980.
26. Dunlap LB, Oregon E: A modified, simple device for the emergency administration of percutaneous transtracheal ventilation. *JACEP* 7:42, 1978.
27. Smith RB, Schaer WB, Pfaeffle H: Percutaneous transtracheal ventilation for anaesthesia and resuscitation: A review and report of complications. *Can Anaesth Soc J* 22:607, 1975.

Vascular Access

Establishing vascular access for infusing medications and fluids and obtaining blood specimens for laboratory examination is a crucial step in pediatric advanced life support. While the intratracheal route is an alternative for the emergency administration of some medications, intravenous or intraosseous access is mandatory for the infusion of fluids, especially when cardiopulmonary arrest results from noncardiac causes such as trauma or sepsis. Arterial cannulation provides a direct means of measuring blood pressure and for obtaining blood samples for oxygen and acid–base analysis and is useful for monitoring the progress of the resuscitation efforts. This chapter reviews percutaneous techniques for intravenous, intraosseous, and intraarterial cannulation and surgical cannulation of the saphenous vein in infants and children.

I. Venous Cannulation

A. General Principles

During cardiopulmonary resuscitation, the largest and most easily accessible vein that does not require the interruption of resuscitation is the preferred access site.

Central cannulation allows the use of a larger cannula and is a more direct route for drug administration than peripheral cannulation. Central access can be obtained via the femoral, internal jugular, external jugular, and, in older children, subclavian veins. The femoral vein is often used because it is relatively easily cannulated without interfering with the resuscitation effort.

Peripheral venipuncture can be performed in veins of the scalp, arm, hand, leg, and foot.[1] It has the disadvantage of small vessel size and distance from the central circulation.

In the course of cardiopulmonary resuscitation, large volumes of fluid, given inadvertently, may cause post-resuscitation complications. In order to avoid this hazard, infusion pumps should be used for all intravenous infusions in infants and children except when large volumes are deliberately given as part of the resuscitation effort. If infusion pumps are not available, mini-drip chambers should be used and the infusion rate carefully regulated by gravity.

B. Complications

Complications of intravascular access procedures include hematoma formation, cellulitis, thrombosis, phlebitis, pulmonary thromboembolism, air embolism, and catheter-fragment embolism.[2] If venous access is attempted in the head and neck, ventilations and chest compressions frequently must be interrupted.

C. Cannulae

Four types of venous cannulae are used in infants and children: 1) butterfly needles, 2) over-the-needle catheters, 3) through-the-needle catheters, and 4) catheter-introducing sheaths.

1. Butterfly Needles

Butterfly needles are useful in obtaining blood specimens for laboratory analysis but, because they tend to infiltrate easily, should not be used for primary venous access during CPR. They have been superceded by over-the-needle catheters.

2. Over-the-Needle Catheters

Over-the-needle catheters can be inserted into veins on the dorsum of the hands and feet, the antecubital fossa, as well as the external jugular and saphenous veins. A variety of sizes is available (Table 4.1); the smallest — 24 gauge — may be used in premature infants. Over-the-needle catheters may also be introduced into the femoral vein for initial resuscitation prior to the introduction of a longer catheter.

3. Through-the-Needle Catheters

Access to the central venous circulation can be obtained via the internal jugular, external jugular, subclavian, and femoral veins with through-the-needle catheters. In children, a 19-gauge catheter (17-gauge needle) or a 16-gauge catheter (14-gauge needle) provides a wide bore for rapid administration of drugs or fluids. In infants, a 22-gauge catheter (19-gauge needle) is relatively easier to place than a larger size; but its small diameter precludes rapid volume expansion. Great care must be exercised with a through-the-needle catheter to prevent its being sheared off by the sharp needle. If any difficulties are encountered in advancing the catheter, it should not be withdrawn through the needle. To prevent catheter-fragment embolization, the entire assembly should be withdrawn as a unit.

4. Pressure-Monitoring Catheters and Catheter-Introducing Sheaths

The Seldinger technique is especially useful in small children as it allows the introduction of large catheters (Table 4.1) into the central venous circulation after initial venous entry with a small-gauge needle or an over-the-needle catheter. When there is free flow of blood, a guide-wire is threaded through the needle or catheter into the

Table 4.1 Equipment for Venous Cannulation

Age (yr.)	Weight (kg)	Butterfly Needles (gauge)	Over-the-Needle Catheters (gauge)	Intracaths Catheter (gauge)	Intracaths Needle (gauge)	Venous Catheters French Size	Venous Catheters Length (cm)	Venous Catheters Wire Diam. [mm (in.)]	Venous Catheters Needle (gauge)	Catheter Introducers French Size	Catheter Introducers Length (cm)	Catheter Introducers Wire Diam. [mm (in.)]	Catheter Introducers Needle (gauge)
<1	<10	21, 23, 25	20, 22, 24	22	19	3.0	8	0.46 (.018)	21	4.0	6	0.53 (.021)	20
										4.5	6	0.53 (.021)	20
1-12	10-40	16, 18, 20	16, 18, 20	18	16	4.0	12	0.53 (.021)	20	5.0	13	0.64 (.025)	19
										5.5	13	0.64 (.025)	19
										6.5	13	0.64 (.025)	19
>12	>40	16, 18, 20	14, 16, 18	16	14	5.0	20	0.89 (.035)	18	7.0	13	0.89 (.035)	18
						6.0	20		18	8.0	13	0.89 (.035)	18

vessel and the needle (or catheter) is removed. A long pressure-monitoring catheter or an introducing sheath is then passed over the wire into the vessel. A catheter-introducing sheath consists of a dilator inside a sheath, both of which are passed over the guidewire. When the guidewire and dilator are removed, the large-bore sheath can be used for infusing fluids or inserting a catheter into the central venous circulation.

D. Cannulation of Peripheral Veins

1. Sites

Scalp Veins: The major superficial veins of the scalp are the frontal, superficial temporal, posterior auricular, supraorbital, occipital, and posterior facial. These small veins are rarely useful during resuscitation efforts but are useful for the administration of fluids and medications after stabilization.

Upper Extremity: The cephalic, median basilic, and median antecubital veins in the forearm may be difficult to locate in chubby babies (Figure 4.1). In the dorsum of the hand, the commonly used veins include tributaries of the cephalic and basilic veins, as well as the dorsal venous arch.

Lower Extremity: The saphenous veins, the median marginal veins, and the veins of the dorsal arch of the lower extremities may all be accessible for cannulation (Figure 4.2).

2. Technique

For Scalp Veins:
1. Restrain the patient.
2. Shave the selected site and surrounding skin.
3. Place a rubberband tourniquet around the head.
4. Clean skin overlying the vein with an antiseptic solution.
5. Check the patency of a butterfly needle or an over-the-needle catheter by injecting sterile solution through the system.
6. Disconnect the syringe from the needle or catheter but leave fluid in the system.
7. Stretch the skin over the vein and identify the direction of blood flow.

8. Introduce the needle through the skin; advance it into the vein until blood flows back freely.
9. Remove the tourniquet.
10. Test the position of the needle by introducing a small amount of sterile solution.
11. Tape needle in place.
12. Evacuate any air in the connecting tubing and attach the infusion.

For Upper or Lower Extremities:
1. Immobilize extremity to be used and stretch the vein. For antecubital fossa veins, place a soft roll of gauze behind the elbow to hyperextend it; for the hand veins, hold the hand firmly with the wrist flexed.
2. Use a cannula (Table 4.1) with an inner stylette needle and a clear hub in order to see blood flashback immediately.
3. Flush the cannula with sterile saline.
4. Apply a tourniquet proximal to the vein.
5. If time permits, puncture the skin slightly distal to the proposed venipuncture site with an 18- or 20-gauge needle to faciliate entry of the cannula.
6. Insert the cannula with the stylette into the vein with the bevel of the needle down.
7. Slowly advance the needle a few millimeters further.
8. Advance the cannula into the vessel and remove the stylette.

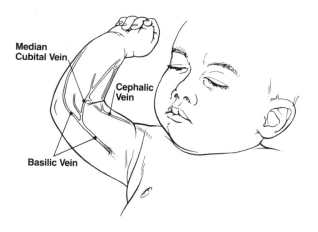

Median Cubital Vein

Cephalic Vein

Basilic Vein

Figure 4.1. Veins of the upper extremity.

9. Check for the free flow of blood from the cannula, tape it in place, attach an infusion set, and apply an antibiotic ointment to the insertion site.

E. Cannulation of Central Veins

Central venous cannulation offers the advantages of a rapid delivery of infusate, the delivery of medications closer to their site of action, and the ability to measure central venous pressure.

Central venous pressure not only depends on the circulating blood volume but also is a reflection of myocardial function and venous compliance, and it is influenced by positive-pressure ventilation and the presence of pneumothorax. It is measured with a catheter in the right atrium or at its junction with the superior or inferior vena cava, with the zero reference point at the level of the mid-right atrium (normal values are 1–5 mmHg or 1–7 cmH$_2$O). Inferior cava pressure may not accurately reflect central venous pressure because it is influenced by the intraabdominal pressure.

Complications of central venous cannulation include infection, hemorrhage, pneumothorax, hemothorax, hydrothorax, cardiac tamponade, air embolism, and catheter-fragment embolism. These hazards are more common in the pediatric age group, and care should be taken to ensure that in a particular clinical setting the benefits outweigh the risks. An experienced operator should perform or supervise this procedure.

1. Sites

The superior vena cava may be cannulated via the external jugular, the internal jugular, or the subclavian vein. The inferior vena cava is entered through the femoral vein. Of these, the external jugular approach is probably the safest because of the superficial and visible nature of the vein. The femoral vein has the advantages of relative ease of access and the distance from major sites of activity during resuscitation. Its major disadvantage is the possibility of pooling medications in the inferior vena cava during external chest compressions, but this can be overcome by using a long catheter and placing the tip above the diaphragm. Internal jugular and subclavian vein cannulation should be performed only by individuals specifically trained and skilled in the technique.

Through-the-needle catheters frequently do not pass freely from the external jugular vein to the superior vena cava due to the acute angle at the junction of the superior vena cava with the subclavian vein. Catheters placed over a J wire by the Seldinger technique are more easily passed into the superior vena cava. In children, a 10- to 14-cm catheter is used, and the distance for advancing the catheter is approximated from surface measurements.

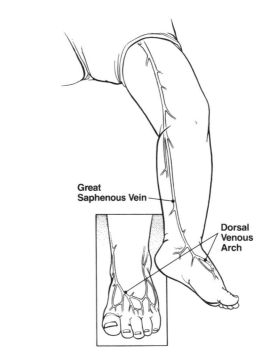

Figure 4.2. Veins of the lower extremity.

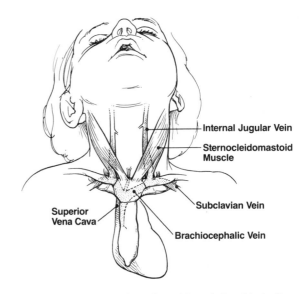

Figure 4.3. The internal jugular vein and its relationship to the surrounding anatomy.

The anatomy of the internal jugular vein and its relation to the sternocleidomastoid muscle and the clavicle are shown in Figure 4.3. Despite the potential hazards, cannulation of this vein can be performed successfully, even in newborns, with training and experience. Three approaches are possible:[3] the posterior, the central (middle), and the anterior routes. Data comparing the success and complication rates of these approaches are not conclusive. Rao[4] described an approach through the central route in which the internal jugular vein is entered just

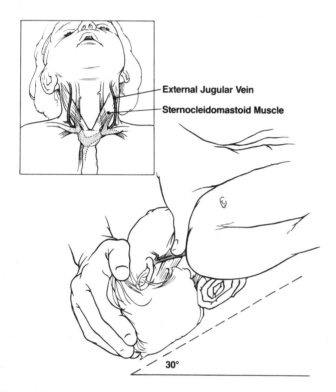

External Jugular Vein

Sternocleidomastoid Muscle

30°

Figure 4.4. External jugular vein technique.

above the clavicle (low approach) rather than at the apex of a triangle formed by the sternal and clavicular bodies of the sternocleidomastoid muscle and the clavicle (high approach). Cote, *et al.,*[5] compared the high and low the central routes and found equal success with each; however, because more complications were associated with the low approach, the high approach was recommended. Prince, *et al.,*[6] described the high central route in detail and had high success and low complication rates. Hall and Geefhuysen[7] and Krausz, *et al.,*[8] studied both the posterior and the central routes, but neither group commented specifically on which route was more successful. The high central approach appears to be the most popular route for entry into the internal jugular vein, but the choice must rest with the experience of the operator.

The Seldinger technique affords excellent access into the central venous system via the femoral vein during an acute emergency.

2. Technique

For the External Jugular Vein: (See Figure 4.4.)
1. Place the child in a 20–30° Trendelenburg position with the head turned away from the side to be punctured. The right side is preferred.
2. Restrain the child.
3. Identify the external jugular vein.
4. Scrub the skin with an antiseptic solution.
5. Wash your hands and wear sterile gloves.

6. Anesthetize the skin with 1% lidocaine.
7. Make an entry point through the skin with a 16- or 18-gauge needle, but do not enter the vein.
8. Insert an over-the-needle catheter into the vein for peripheral cannulation. Insert a through-the-needle catheter or catheter-over-guidewire for central cannulation.
9. When free flow of blood is obtained, make sure that no air bubbles are present in the tubing and attach an infusion set.
10. Suture or tape the catheter firmly in place.
11. Obtain a chest x-ray to ensure that the catheter tip is in the correct position (superior vena cava and right atrium junction).

For the Internal Jugular Vein: The following technique is common to all three routes (i.e., posterior, anterior, and central) of internal jugular vein cannulation (Figure 4.5). The right side of the neck is preferred in children because 1) the dome of the right lung and pleura is lower than the left, 2) the path to the right atrium is more direct, and 3) there is less risk of damage to the thoracic duct.

1. Restrain the infant or child in a 20–45° Trendelenburg position with the head turned to the contralateral side of the venipuncture site.
2. Hyperextend the patient's head by placing a towel roll under the shoulders.
3. Identify the anatomical landmarks of the sternocleidomastoid muscle and the clavicle.
4. Scrub the skin overlying the venipuncture site with an antiseptic solution.
5. Wash your hands and wear sterile gloves.
6. Anesthetize the skin overlying the venipuncture site with 1% lidocaine.
7. Introduce a hollow needle into the vein (see below for specific technique) while applying gentle negative pressure to an attached syringe. Once the vein is entered, remove the syringe and place a finger over the needle hub so as to prevent the aspiration of air. During a positive-pressure breath or spontaneous exhalation, advance a guidewire or catheter to the junction of the superior vena cava and right atrium, the distance having been previously determined from surface landmarks. If a guidewire has been used, remove the needle and pass a catheter or catheter-introducing sheath over the wire. Secure the catheter or introducer in place and attach an infusion set. Lower the IV reservoir below head level and allow blood to flow back freely into the IV tubing before starting the infusion. If blood does not flow back freely, assume that the catheter is not in the vessel and remove it.
8. Secure the catheter with suture material and apply antibiotic ointment and dressing.
9. Obtain a chest x-ray to verify catheter position.

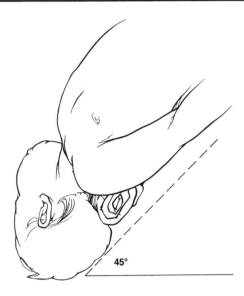

Figure 4.5. The Trendelenburg position for internal jugular vein puncture.

The specific techniques for each of the three internal jugular vein routes used for cannulation follow below. Becoming familiar with one technique rather than randomly attempting all three is recommended.

1. Posterior Route: Introduce the needle under the sternocleidomastoid muscle at the junction of the middle and lower thirds of the posterior margin or just above the point where the external jugular vein crosses this muscle. Aim the needle at the suprasternal notch (Figure 4.6A).

2. Anterior Route: On the right side, retract the carotid artery medially away from the anterior border of the sternocleidomastoid muscle with your index and third fingers. Introduce the needle at the midpoint of this anterior border at a 30–45° angle with the coronal plane. Direct the needle caudally in the sagittal plane toward the ipsilateral nipple (Figure 4.6B).

3. Central Route: Identify a triangle formed by the two portions of the sternocleidomastoid muscle with the clavicle at its base. Insert the needle caudally at the apex of this triangle at a 30° angle to the coronal plane and direct it toward the ipsilateral nipple. If the vein is not entered, direct the needle more laterally toward the ipsilateral shoulder (Figure 4.6C).

A

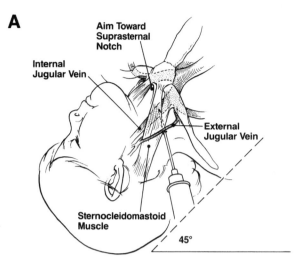

B

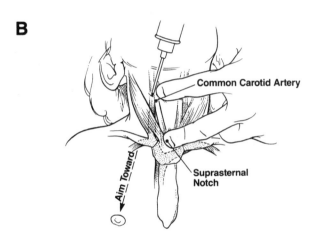

C

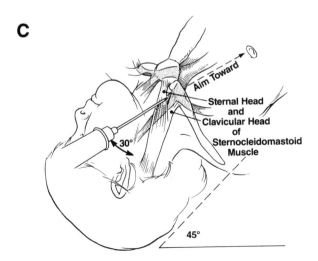

Figure 4.6. Internal jugular vein technique. (A) posterior route; (B) anterior route; (C) central route.

For the Femoral Vein: (See Figure 4.7A and B.)

1. Restrain the leg with slight external rotation.
2. Identify the femoral artery by palpation or, if pulsations are absent, by finding the midpoint between the anterior superior iliac spine and the symphysis pubis.
3. Scrub the area thoroughly with an antiseptic solution.
4. Wash hands and wear sterile gloves.
5. Anesthetize the skin with 1% lidocaine.
6. Puncture the skin with a hollow needle one finger's breadth below the inguinal ligament and just medial to the femoral artery. During chest compressions, pulsations in the femoral area are as likely to originate from the femoral vein as from the artery,[9] and needle puncture should be attempted at the point of pulsation. Direct the needle cephalad at a 45° angle and advance it slowly until a free flow of blood is obtained. Insert the through-the-needle catheter or catheter-introducing sheath as previously described. Remove the needle, or guidewire and dilator, and secure.

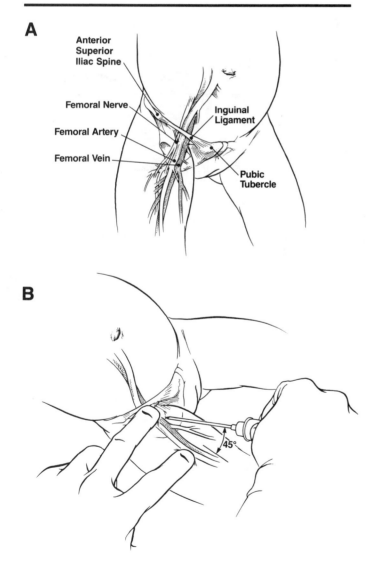

A

Anterior Superior Iliac Spine

Femoral Nerve

Femoral Artery

Femoral Vein

Inguinal Ligament

Pubic Tubercle

B

45°

Figure 4.7. Femoral vein (A) anatomy and (B) technique.

For the Subclavian Vein: Subclavian vein entry into the central venous circulation can be performed in infants and children by the infraclavicular route[10] but has been accompanied by a high rate of complications when performed during emergencies.[11] For this reason it is not recommended for small children unless alternate routes are not available. It may be used safely in older children. (See Figure 4.8A and B.)

1. Place the child in a 20–30° Trendelenburg position with the head turned away from the side to be punctured.
2. Restrain the child.
3. Identify the junction of the middle and medial thirds of the clavicle.
4. Scrub the skin with an antiseptic solution.
5. Wash your hands and wear sterile gloves.
6. Anesthetize the skin with 1% lidocaine.
7. Introduce a needle attached to a syringe just under the clavicle at the junction of the middle and medial thirds of the clavicle and direct it toward a fingertip placed in the suprasternal notch. The syringe and needle should be parallel to the frontal plane, directed medially and slightly cephalad, behind the clavicle toward the posterior superior aspect of the sternal end of the clavicle (the lower end of the fingertip in the sternal notch).
8. Apply gentle suction with the syringe plunger while advancing the needle. When the lumen of the needle enters the vein, rotate the bevel caudally 90° (clockwise) to facilitate placement of the catheter or guidewire into the superior vena cava.
9. When a free flow of blood is obtained, disconnect the syringe and occlude the hub of the needle with a finger to prevent the aspiration of air.
10. During a positive-pressure ventilation or a spontaneous exhalation, insert a guidewire into the vessel and advance it to the superior vena cava, the distance having previously been determined from surface landmarks.
11. Remove the needle and insert a catheter-introducing sheath. Remove the guidewire and introducer.
12. Secure the catheter or introducing sheath; apply antibiotic ointment and sterile dressing.

II. Saphenous Vein Cutdown

If peripheral or central venous cannulation is not obtainable, a saphenous vein cutdown is performed. It may be a particularly valuable alternative in patients above the age of 3 years with hypovolemic shock.

Technique: The long saphenous vein courses anterior to the medial malleolus at the ankle (Figure 4.9). Identify a point (proposed incision site) one finger's breadth superior and anterior to the medial malleolus in children and one-half finger's breadth anterior and superior in infants. The following technique is then used.

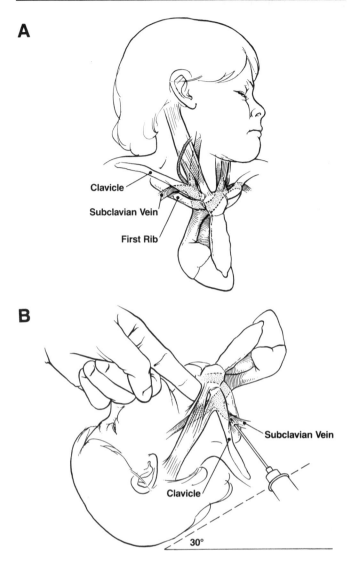

Figure 4.8. Subclavian vein. (A) anatomy and (B) technique.

1. Apply a tourniquet proximal to the proposed incision site.
2. If time permits, scrub skin with an antiseptic solution.
3. Wash your hands, wear sterile gloves, and drape the area with a sterile drape.
4. Infiltrate the overlying skin with 1% lidocaine and make an incision perpendicular to the long axis of the tibia through the skin and subcutaneous tissue.
5. Pass a small curved hemostat, with the tips up, down to the bone, spread the tips, and bring it up from the incision site. The saphenous vein should be picked up by the hemostat. Alternatively, the subcutaneous tissue may be dissected with the tips of the hemostat to identify the saphenous vein before elevating it.
6. Once the vein has been isolated, tie a suture on the distal end of the vein and anchor the vein in place using the tie.

7. Make a venotomy through the vein with a No. 11 scalpel blade inserted perpendicular to the long axis of the vessel into the upper third of the vessel. Thread a cannula or catheter into the vein opening. Tie the proximal suture to hold the catheter in place, and tie the distal suture around the catheter.
8. Remove the tourniquet, suture the incision site, and dress it with antiseptic ointment and sterile dressing.

III. Intraosseous Cannulation

Rossetti, et al.,[12,13] have documented the difficulty in rapidly obtaining vascular access in children, especially those under two years of age, in emergency situations. The intraosseous administration of fluids and medications has long been known to be a safe and effective procedure in children under six years of age. Catecholamines,[14] whole blood, calcium, antibiotics, digitalis, heparin, lidocaine, atropine, and sodium bicarbonate have been successfully infused by the intraosseous route. Meola[15] reported 326 successful bone marrow infusions with only one complication. Heinild, et al.,[16] reported the results of 984 infusions of over two days' duration. Five children developed osteomyelitis, the only complication, but none of these were in patients receiving isotonic fluid. Intraosseous fluid and drug administration would therefore appear to be a valuable and safe technique in the treatment of critically ill infants and children and should be considered as a temporary measure during emergencies when other vascular sites are not immediately available.[17,18]

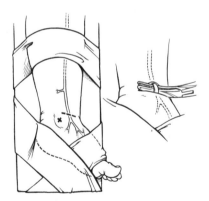

Figure 4.9. Saphenous vein cutdown.

Technique. A standard 16- or 18-gauge hypodermic needle, spinal needle with stylette, bone marrow needle, or trephin is inserted into the anterior surface of the tibial bone 1–3 cm below the tibial tuberosity. The needle should be directed perpendicularly or slightly inferiorly in order to avoid the epiphyseal plate (Figure 4.10). Berg[14] points out that the infusion will be successful if the needle is clearly in the marrow cavity as evidenced by 1) a lack of resistance after the needle passes through the bony cortex, 2) the needle standing upright without support, 3) the ability to aspirate bone marrow into a syringe connected to the needle, and 4) free flow of the infusion without significant subcutaneous infiltration. If the needle becomes obstructed with bone or marrow, it can be replaced with a second needle passed through the same cannulation site.

IV. Priorities in Venous Access

Because intravenous access may be extremely difficult in infants and small children, a protocol is needed to prioritize access for administering drugs and fluids during resuscitation (Figure 4.11). Kanter, *et al.*,[19] have evaluated one such protocol and found that vascular access was obtained sooner when the protocol was used (median, 4.5 minutes) than when it was not used (median, 10 minutes).

Medications, including epinephrine, atropine, lidocaine, and naloxone, should be administered via the endotracheal tube while vascular access is being established. In children under 6 years of age, an intraosseous cannula should be placed immediately and used for volume expansion and additional medications. In older children (6 years or older) vascular access should be obtained by a cutdown over the saphenous vein or a central route, the choice depending on the skill of the rescuers. Of the central venous access sites, the femoral is probably the safest and easiest to cannulate.

V. Arterial Cannulation

Following restoration of spontaneous circulation, arterial access is helpful in monitoring blood pressure and evaluating the adequacy of ventilation/oxygenation. Indwelling

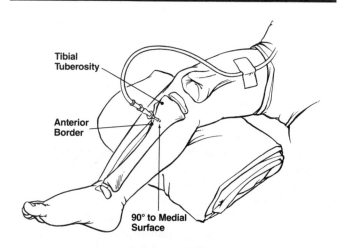

Figure 4.10. Intraosseous cannulation technique.

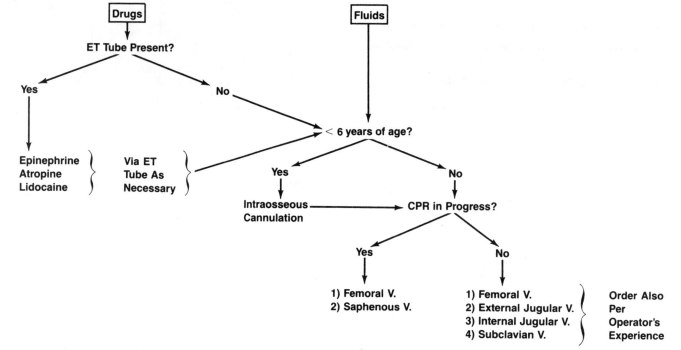

Attempt Peripheral Venous Access.
If not immediately successful and vascular access required for

Figure 4.11. Priorities for vascular access.

arterial catheters can be placed percutaneously in the radial, femoral, dorsalis pedis, and posterior tibial arteries. Temporal artery cannulation may be associated with severe cerebral thromboembolic complications, perhaps caused by migration of thrombus to the internal carotid circulation, and is best avoided.[20,21]

A modified Allen test, to assess the adequacy of collateral flow from the ulnar artery, must be performed before radial artery cannulation. The hand of the infant or child is passively clenched and compressed while pressure is maintained on both the ulnar and the radial arteries. The pressure on the ulnar artery is released: If the entire hand flushes while the radial artery remains occluded, flow from the ulnar artery is considered adequate. A similar test should be performed to demonstrate adequacy of flow to the foot prior to cannulation of the dorsalis pedis artery. The dorsalis pedis artery is occluded and the big toe is blanched by compressing the toenail for several seconds. The pressure on the nail is released: A rapid return of color indicates adequate collateral flow.

A. Radial Artery Technique

A fiberoptic light placed under the wrist of small infants has been found to be helpful in locating the radial artery.[22] (See Figure 4.12A and B.)

1. Dorsiflex the hand at the wrist to 45–60° and secure both the hand and the lower forearm to a board. A roll of gauze behind the wrist will maintain dorsiflexion. Tape the hand, leaving all fingers exposed so that the adequacy of circulation can be assessed.

2. Locate the radial artery just proximal to the head of the radius.
3. Scrub the overlying skin with an antiseptic solution.
4. Wash your hands, wear sterile gloves, and drape the area with sterile towels.
5. Anesthetize the skin with 1% lidocaine without epinephrine.
6. Puncture the skin at the site of maximal pulsation with a 20-gauge needle or a No. 11 blade held parallel to the skin. Advance a 22-gauge, 1-inch, heparin-flushed Teflon catheter into the puncture site at a 30° angle and advance it until blood appears in the hub. Two techniques have been used successfully in catheter placement:
   a. Pass the catheter and needle through the artery to transfix it. Withdraw the needle, and then withdraw the catheter very slowly until there is free flow of blood. Now advance the catheter slowly through the lumen of the artery.
   b. Puncture only the anterior wall of the artery. Advance the catheter slowly until blood appears in the needle. Lower the needle carefully to a 10° angle; ascertain that blood flow is continuing. Advance the catheter slowly over the needle into the lumen of the artery.
7. Remove the needle and attach the catheter to a T-connector to permit continuous infusion of heparinized isotonic saline (1 U/mL).
8. Cover the puncture site with antibiotic ointment, a pressure dressing, and adhesive tape.
9. Remove gauze roll and secure the wrist in a neutral position to the board.

B. Complications

The use of indwelling arterial catheters is accompanied by the risk of localized or generalized infection, air or particulate embolization, inadvertent injection of a sclerosing solution, and thrombosis of the artery. Miyasaka[23] reported the complications in 53 consecutive arterial cannulations in 47 pediatric patients. The most common problems were skin lesions, usually insignificant; localized necrosis (34%) and occlusion of the radial artery (50%) were also seen. Predisposing factors for occlusion of the radial artery were 1) age of the patient (66% in children younger than 5 years of age vs. 34% in those more than 5 years of age), 2) insertion technique (70% in those with a cutdown vs. 31% in those with a percutaneous technique), and 3) duration of cannulation (71% in those greater than 4 days vs. 44% in those less than 4 days).

A
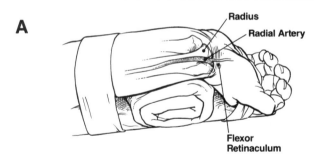

B
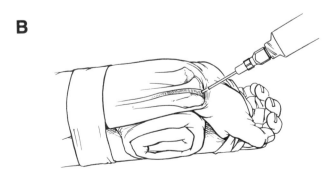

Figure 4.12. Radial artery (A) anatomy and (B) technique.

References

1. Filston HC, Johnson DG: Percutaneous venous cannulation in neonates and infants: A method for catheter insertion without "cut down." *Pediatrics* 48:896, 1971.
2. Kaye W: Catheter and infusion-related sepsis: The nature of the problem and its prevention, in *Textbook of Advanced Cardiac Life Support,* Dallas, AHA, 1983.
3. DeFalque RJ: Percutaneous catheterization of the internal jugular vein. *Anesth Analg* 53:116, 1974.
4. Rao TL, Wong AY, Salem MR: A new approach to percutaneous catheterization of the internal jugular vein. *Anesthesiology* 46:362, 1977.
5. Cote CJ, Jobes DR, Schwartz AJ, et al.: Two approaches to cannulation of a child's internal jugular vein. *Anesthesiology* 50:371, 1979.
6. Prince SR, Sullivan RL, Hackel A: Percutaneous catheterization of the internal jugular vein in infants and children. *Anesthesiology* 44:170, 1976.
7. Hall DM, Geefhuysen J: Percutaneous catheterization of the internal jugular vein in infants and children. *J Pediatr Surg* 12:719, 1977.
8. Krausz MM, Berlatzky YB, Ayalon A, et al: Percutaneous cannulation of the internal jugular vein in infants and children. *Surg Gynecol Obstet* 148:591, 1979.
9. Niemann JT, Rosborough JP, Ung S, et al: Hemodynamic effects of continuous abdominal binding during cardiac arrest and resuscitation. *Am J Cardiol* 53:269, 1984.
10. Filston HC, Grant JP: A safer system for percutaneous subclavian venous catheterization in newborn infants. *J Pediatr Surg* 14:564, 1979.
11. Groff DB, Ahmed N: Subclavian vein catheterization in the infant. *J Pediatr Surg* 9:171, 1974.
12. Rossetti V, Thompson BM, Aprahamian C, et al: Difficulty and delay in intravascular access in pediatric arrests, abstracted. *Ann Emerg Med* 13:406, 1984.
13. Rossetti VA, Thompson BM, Miller J, et al: Intraosseous infusions: An alternative route of pediatric intravascular access. *Ann Emerg Med* 14:885, 1985.
14. Berg RA: Emergency infusion of catecholamines into bone marrow. *Am J Dis Child* 138:810, 1984.
15. Meola F: Bone marrow infusions as routine procedure in children. *J Pediatr* 25:13, 1944.
16. Heinild S, Sondergaard T, Tudvad F: Bone marrow infusion in childhood: Experiences from 1,000 infusions. *J Pediatr* 30:400, 1947.
17. McNamara RM, Spivey WH, Sussman C: Pediatric resuscitation without an intravenous line. *Am J Emerg Med* 4:31, 1986.
18. Glaeser PW, Losek JD: Emergency intraosseous infusions in children. *Am J Emerg Med* 4:34, 1986.
19. Kanter RK, Zimmerman JJ, Strauss RN, et al: Pediatric emergency intravenous access: Evaluation of a protocol. *Am J Dis Child* 140:132, 1986.
20. Simmons MA, Levine RL, Lubchenco LO, et al: Warning: Serious sequelae of temporal artery catheterization. *J Pediatr* 92:284, 1978.
21. Bull MJ, Schreiner RL, Garg BP, et al: Neurologic complications following temporal artery catheterizations. *J Pediatr* 96:1071, 1980.
22. Cole FS, Todres ID, Shannon DC: Technique for percutaneous cannulation of the radial artery in the newborn infant. *J Pediatr* 92:105, 1978.
23. Miyasaka K, Edmonds JF, Conn AW: Complications of radial artery lines in the pediatric patient. *Can Anaesth Soc J* 23:9, 1976.

Fluid Therapy and Medications
(For Optional Drug Therapy Chapter, See Appendix D)

The actions and clinical indications of medications essential for the resuscitation of infants and children suffering from cardiac arrest are reviewed in this chapter. It includes discussions of fluid therapy and acid–base balance and, for each medication, therapeutic considerations, indications, dosages, routes of administration, precautions, and the clinically recommended available forms.

The objectives of medications used during cardiac arrest are:

1. to correct hypoxemia;
2. to increase perfusion pressure during chest compression;
3. to stimulate spontaneous or more forceful myocardial contraction;
4. to accelerate the cardiac rate;
5. to correct metabolic acidosis; and
6. to suppress ventricular ectopy.

I. Volume Expansion

Hypovolemic shock (discussed in Chapter 1) is a common problem in pediatric patients who require emergency care. This is particularly true following trauma and burns but may also result from diarrhea with dehydration, diabetic ketoacidosis, and vomiting with poor intake. Septic shock, although not usually classified as hypovolemic, is characterized by relative hypovolemia due to vasodilation from a decrease in vascular tone. The initial emergency therapies of these two forms of shock are similar and require vascular access (see Chapter 4). In traumatic (i.e., hemorrhagic) shock, since large volumes of blood and fluid are needed, the largest bore, short intravascular cannula should be inserted and at least two secure lines should be established.

The type of fluid used for initial volume expansion is controversial. Crystalloid solutions, such as lactated Ringer's solution and normal saline, are inexpensive, readily available, and free from allergic reactions. They effectively expand the interstitial water space and correct sodium deficits, but they are not efficient in expanding the circulating volume. Since only about one fourth of the infused crystalloid solution remains in the plasma compartment, four to five times the deficit must be infused to restore plasma volume. In healthy young patients this quantity is well tolerated, but in the critically ill child with underlying cardiac or pulmonary disease, it may lead to pulmonary edema.

Blood and colloids, such as 5% albumin, fresh frozen plasma, and the synthetic colloids (Hetastarch, Dextran 40, Dextran 60), are much more efficient in rapidly expanding the intravascular compartment, and at least

one of these should be readily available. Major disadvantages include potential adverse reactions and higher cost.

With either type of fluid, a frequent error in fluid resuscitation from hypovolemic shock in children is in not providing adequate volume replacement. The principle of fluid therapy is to give a volume bolus, reassess the patient, then give additional boluses with frequent reassessment. The assessment signs discussed in Chapter 1 include skin color and warmth, volume and quality of peripheral pulses, mental status, heart rate, and urine output. Note that blood pressure is not mentioned. Children often present with normal blood pressure despite the presence of other signs of shock. Early recognition and treatment of shock are essential to avoid hypotension; if the latter occurs, resuscitation is more difficult.

Hypovolemic shock results from a depleted intravascular as well as extravascular volume space. Depending on the degree and duration of the deficit, the microvasculature loses normal tone and the capillaries become more permeable. Volume administration in excess of estimated losses is necessary since fluid is lost from transcapillary leakage and the loss of vascular tone expands the vascular compartment, which must be filled.

In the patient with hypovolemic shock, 20 mL/kg of crystalloid solution should be given as soon as vascular access is obtained. Ringer's lactate may be preferred since it avoids hyperchloremic acidosis that may result from the infusion of large volumes of sodium chloride. Large volumes of dextrose-containing solutions are best not given unless hypoglycemia is documented, since the resulting hyperglycemia may induce an osmotic diuresis. Blood should be given to traumatic shock victims as soon as it is available in order to replace blood loss. Blood administration may also be helpful in septic and other forms of shock, but it is not a first-line volume expander in these settings. The crystalloid bolus is given as rapidly as possible (in less than 20 minutes). A three-way stopcock attached to a 20- or 50-mL syringe may be useful in facilitating rapid volume infusion. The child is then reassessed, and if perfusion is still diminished, an additional 20 mL/kg of volume is given. Subsequent volume may be either colloid or crystalloid and is given as needed, based on repeated reassessment of the patient. A child with hypovolemic shock often requires at least 40–60 mL/kg in the first hour of resuscitation, and occasionally, up to 100–200 mL/kg may be needed in the first few hours. In septic shock, at least 60–80 mL/kg is often required in the first hour. The key to successful fluid therapy is frequent patient reassessment and the infusion of a sufficient amount of fluid. However, beware that in the seriously or multiply injured child, volume losses due to continuing hemorrhage, especially when hypotension is present, may be ongoing. In most such cases, volume expansion alone is not sufficient to restore effective circulation, and immediate surgical help must be obtained.

II. General Guidelines for Administering Medications

During a cardiac arrest, intravenous access is preferred for drug administration, but since it may be difficult to achieve,[1] the endotracheal route can be used to deliver atropine, epinephrine, naloxone, and lidocaine.[2] Optimal endotracheal doses for pediatric patients are not known. Although studies suggest that a larger dose must be given endotracheally than intravenously to produce the same hemodynamic effects,[3,4] in the absence of data in children, at least the same dose given intravenously is recommended for endotracheal administration. Medications must be injected as deeply as possible into the tracheobronchial tree in order to be absorbed.[5] This is best achieved by injecting the medication, diluted in 1–2 mL of normal saline, through a catheter passed beyond the endotracheal tube tip, followed by several positive-pressure ventilations.

Central venous administration of medications during external chest compressions provides more rapid onset and higher peak concentrations than peripheral venous injection.[6] In adult animal models, injection into the central supradiaphragmatic venous system achieves better drug delivery into the circulation than intravenous injection below the diaphragm.[7] It is uncertain whether the site of injection is as important in the infant or small child, and either site is acceptable.

Medications, including catecholamines, are well absorbed from the bone marrow[8,9] (see Chapter 4); intraosseous injection can therefore be considered equivalent to intravenous injection and is preferable to the endotracheal route in children under 6 years of age. Following the injection of medications, the intravascular line should be flushed with 1–2 mL of normal saline in an infant and 5 mL in the older child to speed delivery into the central circulation. Small boluses of saline following drug administration are safer than rapid infusions of maintenance intravenous fluid. Caution should be used to avoid excessive volume infusion, which can compromise vital organ blood flow.[10]

If an intravenous, endotracheal, or intraosseous route is not available, resuscitation medications (epinephrine, sodium bicarbonate, and atropine) may be injected directly into the heart. Intracardiac injections are discouraged, however, because they are associated with significant hazards, including interruption of chest compressions, coronary laceration, cardiac tamponade, and intractable arrhythmias.

Catecholamines (i.e., epinephrine, dopamine, dobutamine, isoproterenol) may be diluted in a number of intravenous solutions: D_5W, $D_{10}W$, $D_5W\frac{1}{2}NS$, D_5NS, or Ringer's lactate for continuous infusion. In the arrest setting, catecholamine infusions should be started rapidly (10–20 mL/hr) until an effect is achieved (i.e., an increase in heart rate or blood pressure); the rate is then decreased to the desired dose. At the slow infusion rates used in children, failure initially to increase the infusion rate may significantly delay delivery of the medication, i.e., until the dead space in the intravenous tubing and catheter are filled. All of the catecholamines are rapidly metabolized, so decreasing the infusion rate as soon as a physiologic effect is seen will prevent toxicity.

III. Resuscitation Medications

A. Oxygen

1. Therapeutic Considerations

During cardiac arrest, a number of factors contribute to severe progressive hypoxemia and tissue hypoxia. Mouth-to-mouth rescue breathing provides about 16–17% oxygen, which at best results in an alveolar oxygen tension of 80 torr (normal in room air is 104 torr). Since even optimal chest compressions provide only a fraction of the normal cardiac output (25–30% in adults), tissue oxygen delivery is markedly compromised. Additionally, cardiopulmonary resuscitation is accompanied by right-to-left intrapulmonary shunting due to ventilation–perfusion mismatching, which is exacerbated if aspiration or pulmonary edema are present.

2. Indications

In hypoxemic patients, an elevation of arterial oxygen tension increases arterial oxygen content and oxygen delivery to the tissues. If possible, oxygen should be used as an emergency measure in all arrest situations, in any condition in which hypoxemia is suspected, and in any condition of respiratory difficulty that may lead to a cardiac arrest (e.g., severe asthma, croup, epiglottitis, foreign body obstruction). Oxygen should never be withheld during an emergency even if the measured arterial oxygen tension is high, since oxygen delivery to the tissues may still be compromised by a low cardiac output.

3. Dose

The highest available concentration of oxygen available should be used until the child is stabilized (see Chapter 3).

4. Precautions

Concern regarding the toxic effect of oxygen on the lungs and, in premature infants, on the eyes is justified, but 100% oxygen should never be withheld from an infant or child during an emergency. If possible, oxygen should be humidified before delivery.

5. Available Preparations

See Chapter 3.

B. Epinephrine

1. Therapeutic Considerations

Epinephrine (adrenaline) is an endogenous catecholamine with both alpha- and beta-adrenergic-receptor stimulating actions.[11] Alpha-adrenergic actions, characterized by vasoconstriction, especially in the splanchnic, mucosal, and dermal vascular beds, result in an increased systemic vascular resistance and an elevated systolic and diastolic blood pressure. Beta-adrenergic-receptor action produces an increase in myocardial contractility and heart rate and relaxation of the smooth muscle in the skeletal muscle vascular bed and in bronchi.

The pharmacologic actions of epinephrine are complex and dose related, but the large dose used in the arrest situation produces prominent alpha-adrenergic effects in the vascular bed and beta-adrenergic effects on the heart. Reflex circulatory adjustments may alter the direct actions of the drug (e.g., significant elevations of blood pressure may produce reflex bradycardia).

Epinephrine has a long history of successful use in the treatment of cardiac arrest; evidence suggests that the alpha-adrenergic effect (i.e., vasoconstriction) is the most important action of epinephrine when used in this setting.[12] Thus, a pure alpha-adrenergic drug such as methoxamine, which lacks any inotropic effect, is highly effective in resuscitation from electromechanical dissociation.[13] Vasoconstriction elevates blood pressure and coronary perfusion pressure, thus enhancing the delivery of oxygen to the heart; this is the most important action of sympathomimetics in the treatment of cardiac arrest.[14] The following cardiovascular effects can be expected from epinephrine in the dose used during resuscitation:

1. Increased heart rate
2. Increased myocardial contractility
3. Increased systemic vascular resistance
4. Increased blood pressure (due to 2 and 3 above)
5. Increased myocardial oxygen requirements (due to 1, 2, and 3 above)
6. Increased automaticity

Clinically, epinephrine elevates the perfusion pressure generated during chest compressions, improves the contractile state, stimulates spontaneous contraction (e.g., in asystole), and increases the vigor of ventricular fibrillation. The latter appears to enhance the ability to terminate ventricular fibrillation by countershock.

2. Indications

The elevation of coronary perfusion pressure following injection of epinephrine is a beneficial effect applicable to all forms of cardiorespiratory arrest.

The most common rhythm disturbances in pediatric patients are asystole and bradyarrhythmias, often associated with pulselessness (i.e., electromechanical dissociation).[15] In these settings, epinephrine may generate electrical and mechanical activity of the heart. In ventricular fibrillation, which is rare in children, epinephrine is used to render the rhythm more susceptible to electrical defibrillation.

The action of catecholamines is depressed by acidosis;[16] attention to adequate ventilation, circulation, and the correction of metabolic acidosis is therefore important.

3. Dose

The recommended initial dose of epinephrine is 0.01 mg/kg of the 1:10,000 solution (0.1 mL/kg) given by the intravenous or intraosseous route. Epinephrine is well absorbed from the tracheobronchial tree, although when the drug is administered via the endotracheal tube, peak blood levels are less than one tenth of those obtained from equal doses administered intravenously.[17,18]

In the absence of clinical data to dictate the optimal endotracheal dose, experimental models suggest that 0.02–0.03 mg/kg be used, with a minimal recommended dose of 1.0 mL of the 1:10,000 solution.[60,61] Delivery of the drug and improved absorption can be facilitated by dilution of the drug with 1 to 2 mL of normal saline. It may be instilled via a catheter that extends beyond the end of the tube, or directly into the endotracheal tube. This may be followed by several rapid positive-pressure breaths.

4. Precautions

Epinephrine should not be added to a bicarbonate infusion since catecholamines are inactivated by an alkaline solution. Careful monitoring of the patient receiving epinephrine is necessary since side effects may include postresuscitation hypertension and tachyarrhythmias.

5. Available Preparations

It is recommended that prefilled syringes of the 1:10,000 solution be used for cardiac resuscitation. These are available in the following forms:

5 ml (0.1 mg/mL)
10 ml (0.1 mg/mL)

C. Sodium Bicarbonate

During cardiopulmonary arrest, hypoxia-induced anaerobic metabolism results in the generation of lactic acid. This is compounded by ventilatory failure, which causes carbon dioxide retention (hypercapnia) and respiratory acidosis. As a consequence, the acidotic state accompanying the arrest of ventilation and circulation is usually of mixed origin — metabolic and respiratory — and is most effectively evaluated by correct interpretation of arterial blood gas analysis. Arterial oxygen tension (PaO_2), arterial carbon dioxide tension ($PaCO_2$), and hydrogen ion (H^+) concentration (i.e., pH) are directly measured from arterial blood. Although oxygen tension is important in overall oxygen delivery to the tissues, only the pH and $PaCO_2$ are important in acid–base balance interpretation.

Metabolic acids, derived from intermediary metabolism of amino acids, fats, and carbohydrates, are normally excreted by the kidney. During cardiac arrest or low cardiac output states, however, renal perfusion is inadequate and acid excretion is insufficient. In addition, lactic acid is produced during anaerobic metabolism and cannot be metabolized until oxygen delivery to the tissues is restored.

1. Buffer Systems

Acid–base balance is normally maintained by several buffer systems. A buffer is a chemical substance that, by its presence in a solution such as plasma, decreases the change in pH that would otherwise occur following the addition of an acid or a base. Physiologic buffers are usually composed of a weak acid and its alkali salt (e.g., H_2CO_3 and HCO_3^-; H_2PO_4 and HPO_4^-). Note that an acid is a proton (hydrogen ion) donor and a base is a proton acceptor.

The bicarbonate buffer system is the most important system for rapid adjustments of pH; other important buffer systems are proteins, phosphate, and hemoglobin. The bicarbonate:carbonic acid buffer is unique because its acid form (H_2CO_3) is volatile. When the bicarbonate anion reacts with an acid, the CO_2 produced can be removed by ventilation; this provides the potential for complete neutralization of a metabolic acid to its neutral salt. Note, however, that ventilation *must* be adequate to permit the elimination of formed CO_2 by the lungs.

The H^+ concentration in the blood is expressed as the pH, which is the negative logarithm of the H^+ concentration. Therefore, a pH of 2 equals 10^{-2} moles per liter of H^+, or 0.01 mol/L; a pH of 7 is 10^{-7} moles per liter of H^+, or 0.0000001 mol/L.

Another way of expressing H^+ concentration is in nanoequivalents (nEq), where 1 nEq = 10^{-9} Eq/L. One million nanoequivalents are equal to 1 mEq. Nanoequivalents are also useful in defining changes in H^+ concentration. Since the pH is related to the logarithm of the H^+ concentration, similar numeric changes in pH are not associated with equivalent changes in H^+. For example, a pH change from 7.2 to 7.1 occurs with an increase of 17 nEq/L of H^+, whereas a pH change from 7.6 to 7.5 is associated with a H^+ concentration increase of 7 nEq/L. A pH of 7.40 is produced by 40 nEq/L of H^+. Note that decreases in pH are associated with numerically larger changes in H^+ concentration than increases in pH.

It should also be obvious that the magnitude of change in the H^+ concentration is substantially smaller than the quantity of bicarbonate given to correct abnormalities in pH. Changes in H^+ concentration are measured in nanoequivalents per liter, whereas bicarbonate is infused in doses of milliequivalents per kilogram of body weight (10^6 times larger). The apparent discrepancy between the dose of bicarbonate infused and the calculated buffer needed to decrease H^+ concentration is actually a reflec-

tion of the efficiency of the other buffer systems, such as intracellular proteins, hemoglobin, and phosphate, in buffering changes in H^+ concentration.

2. Acidosis and Alkalosis

The normal pH is 7.40, with a range from 7.35 to 7.45. A pH below 7.35 defines acidosis; a pH above 7.45, alkalosis. Alterations of acid–base balance may occur on a respiratory or a metabolic basis. These changes in pH are reflected by changes in the concentration of carbon dioxide and sodium bicarbonate. The relation of pH to these alterations is approximated by

$$pH = \frac{base}{acid} = \frac{HCO_3^-}{H_2CO_3} = \frac{20}{1}$$

Carbonic acid, the denominator in the ratio above, is directly related to the $PaCO_2$: An increase in $PaCO_2$ produces an increase in H_2CO_3, a diminshed ratio, and therefore, a lower pH.

Complicating the interpretation of respiratory or metabolic changes in acid–base balance is the compensation by one system for changes in the other. The patient with shock, poor perfusion, and resulting lactic acidosis with bicarbonate depletion may compensate by hyperventilating to decrease the partial pressure of carbon dioxide ($PaCO_2$). Decreased $PaCO_2$ lowers H_2CO_3, thus maintaining the ratio of base:acid closer to 20 and minimizing changes in pH. The patient would then have a primary metabolic acidosis with a compensatory respiratory alkalosis.

Respiratory-induced alterations of pH are produced through changes in $PaCO_2$; the latter also reflect the ventilatory status of the patient. Normal values of $PaCO_2$ range between 35 and 45 torr (mmHg). As ventilation increases, $PaCO_2$ decreases, lowering H_2CO_3 and increasing the ratio of base:acid, and thus the pH. This is defined as respiratory alkalosis.

$PaCO_2$ above 45 torr defines alveolar hypoventilation and respiratory acidosis, whereas $PaCO_2$ less than 35 torr defines alveolar hyperventilation and respiratory alkalosis. Note that alveolar hypoventilation may be present despite tachypnea because rapid breathing, especially in infants and small children, may be associated with shallow breaths. In this situation each breath or tidal volume is small, with increased dead space ventilation and less effective alveolar ventilation.

3. Blood Gas Interpretation

The therapeutic approach to acid–base disorders is simplified by the application of three "Golden Rules."

Golden Rule I estimates the impact of changes in $PaCO_2$ on the measured pH. This rule states that *an acute change in $PaCO_2$ of 10 torr is associated with an increase or a decrease in pH of 0.08 units.* Thus, as $PaCO_2$ increases 10 torr, pH will fall 0.08 units.

In application, if $PaCO_2$ is 40 torr, the pH will be 7.40 (normal) in the absence of a metabolic acidosis. However, if $PaCO_2$ increases to 50 torr, pH will fall to 7.32, thereby defining hypoventilation and respiratory acidosis. Should $PaCO_2$ fall to 30 torr, the pH will rise to 7.48, thereby defining hyperventilation, or respiratory alkalosis.

To assess the respiratory component of acid–base balance from arterial blood gas analysis, the following steps may be employed:

1. Calculate the amount by which the reported $PaCO_2$ either falls below or exceeds 40 torr.
2. Calculate the pH based on the measured $PaCO_2$, according to Golden Rule I.
3. Compare the measured pH to the calculated pH (Step 2).

If the calculated pH is close to the measured pH, all changes are respiratory. If the measured pH is greater than the calculated pH, it constitutes a metabolic alkalosis; if the measured pH is less than calculated, it constitutes a metabolic acidosis.

Therapy of respiratory acidosis is of primary importance in pediatric CPR. Establishing a secure airway and hyperventilating the patient with 100% O_2 will decrease the $PaCO_2$ and effectively oxygenate and correct the acidosis. Respiratory acidosis is *not* treated with the administration of sodium bicarbonate. For sodium bicarbonate to produce any effective buffering action, ventilation must be adequate to eliminate the carbon dioxide formed from the $HCO_3^- + H^+$ reaction.[19]

Golden Rule II: After the respiratory component has been accounted for, a reasonably accurate method of estimating the degree of the metabolic component (acidosis or metabolic alkalosis) is through the application of Golden Rule II. This rule states that *a pH change of 0.15 units is the result of a base change of 10 mEq/L.* Thus, if the pH increases by 0.15 units, there is an increase in base of 10 mEq/L. Conversely, if pH falls 0.15 units, there is a decrease in base of 10 mEq/L. Stated differently, for every 0.01 unit change in pH that is not due to a change in $PaCO_2$, there is a $2/3$ mEq/L change in the base. Thus, a 0.09 unit decrease in pH results from a 6 mEq/L decrease [$9 \times (2/3)$ mEq/L] in base excess, assuming no change in $PaCO_2$.

"Base excess" is a confusing term that describes the presence (in milliequivalents per liter) in the blood of an excess of base or deficit of fixed acid. Base excess is a positive value when there is an excess of base and a negative value when there is either a deficiency of base or an excess of fixed acid. Fixed acid does not include the volatile carbonic acid. Base excess provides a means of quantifying the amount of base or acid that must be added to the blood to restore normal pH.

An alternative expression for a decrease in base, instead of a "negative base excess," is "base deficit." For example, if the $PaCO_2$ were 50 torr and the pH 7.26, the 10 torr increase of $PaCO_2$ by Golden Rule I would define a respiratory acidosis. The calculated pH would be 7.32. Since the measured pH is 7.26, there is a pH difference of 0.06 units. This defines a base *deficit* of 4 mEq/L

[$6 \times (2/3)$]; thus, a metabolic acidosis, as well as a respiratory acidosis, is present.

The substantial base deficit typically seen in cardiac arrest is due to the loss of bicarbonate ions through the buffering of fixed acids. Bicarbonate is located primarily in the extracellular fluid compartment, which is equal to about 30% of body weight (i.e., $0.3 \times$ body weight).[20] This distribution of bicarbonate is used to determine the treatment of metabolic acidosis.

Golden Rule III is the least helpful rule clinically. It states that *the total body bicarbonate deficit equals the base deficit (mEq/L) × the patient's weight (in kg) × 0.3.* In a 25-kg patient with a $PaCO_2$ of 52 torr and a pH of 7.18, the $PaCO_2$ is increased by 12 torr above normal; therefore, we would expect a pH of 7.30. The unexplained pH difference of 0.12 units (7.30–7.18) must be attributed to a metabolic acidosis with a calculated base deficit of 8 mEq/L [$12 \times (2/3)$]. The respiratory component should be treated by increasing ventilation while the metabolic component can be treated with bicarbonate according to Golden Rule III. Since the base deficit is 8 mEq/L and extracellular fluid equals 30% of body weight, the calculation is $8 \times 25 \times 0.3 = 60$ mEq. Complete correction of the calculated base deficit is not indicated, and one half the calculated dose of bicarbonate is used. Note that this amount (30 mEq) is close to 1 mEq/kg, which is an adequate and quickly calculated dose for the treatment of moderate metabolic acidosis.

Hyperventilation, to correct respiratory acidosis, and treatment of shock, to restore a stable, spontaneous circulation, are the only therapies needed in the treatment of mild-to-moderate metabolic acidosis. In the example above, reducing the $PaCO_2$ to 30 torr by hyperventilation will change the pH to 7.36 in the *absence* of any therapy directed at correcting the metabolic component of the acidosis.

Although pH changes are clinically measured in the blood, intracellular changes in pH may play a more important role in maintaining physiological homeostasis. In cerebrospinal fluid (CSF), changes in $PaCO_2$ will alter CSF pH much more rapidly and profoundly than changes in arterial HCO_3^- concentration.[21] The same phenomenon occurs across cellular membranes; increases in $PaCO_2$ depress cardiac function more than decreases in pH produced by fixed acids.[22] Bicarbonate transiently depresses cardiac function, presumably on the basis of a transient increase in $PaCO_2$ and, therefore, cellular pCO_2, with a depression of intracellular pH.[23] Bicarbonate administration in lactic acidosis has been shown to depress intracellular pH in hepatocytes.[24] These studies emphasize the importance of ventilation in the acute management of the child with acidosis accompanying cardiac arrest or shock.

4. Indications, Dose, Precautions, and Available Preparations

Indications: Since respiratory failure is the major cause of cardiac arrest in the pediatric patient,[25] prompt and efficient ventilation of the lungs is essential for the management of both acidemia and hypoxemia of arrest.[18] The treatment of the metabolic component of the acidosis includes hyperventilation to reduce the partial pressure of CO_2, efforts to increase perfusion, and, if necessary, $NaHCO_3$ infusion. Administration of this drug results in a simple acid–base reaction in which the HCO_3^- ion combines with H^+ ions in the blood and thereby elevates the blood pH:

$$HCO_3^- + H^+ \rightleftharpoons H_2CO_3 \rightleftharpoons CO_2 + H_2O$$

Note that carbon dioxide is formed as H^+ is buffered. Since CO_2 can cross cell membranes more rapidly than bicarbonate, the administration of sodium bicarbonate can transiently worsen intracellular acidosis,[26] resulting in impaired myocardial performance.[23] Recent data demonstrate a fall in cardiac index and blood pressure and a worsening of lactic acidosis after sodium bicarbonate administration in hypoxic lactic acidosis.[27] In view of these potential toxicities, sodium bicarbonate is not indicated in mild-to-moderate metabolic acidosis, especially when due to inadequate circulating volume; the acidosis will resolve with ventilation and volume replacement. In severe acidosis (pH < 7.20) the use of bicarbonate is still controversial. In a cardiac arrest, initial attention should always be focused on securing the airway, hyperventilating the patient, and chest compressions. Following these maneuvers, sodium bicarbonate may be used in the patient with continued cardiac arrest or an unstable hemodynamic state.

Dose: The dose of sodium bicarbonate is a subject of some controversy. It was noted above that pH changes are related to logarithmic changes in H^+ ion concentration; thus, the more severe the metabolic acidosis, the greater the need for buffer therapy. The severity of metabolic acidosis is related to the length of the arrest and is likely to be greater in out-of-hospital arrests than in those occurring in hospitalized patients. If the arrest is observed and brief (1–2 minutes), sodium bicarbonate probably need not be given. Even in a cardiac arrest of long duration such as might occur out-of-hospital or in an unmonitored hospitalized patient, initial attention should still be focused on airway, breathing, and epinephrine administration. If the cardiac arrest continues after the airway is secured, the patient is hyperventilated, chest compressions are initiated, and epinephrine is given, then 1 mEq/kg of sodium bicarbonate may be given via the intravenous or intraosseous route. In a hospitalized patient with a shorter duration of arrest, the initial dose should be 0.5–1.0 mEq/kg, since the degree of acidosis is likely to be less. Further doses of sodium bicarbonate should be based on measurements of arterial pH and $PaCO_2$; however, these values may be misleading since they appear to reflect ventilation as opposed to flow and they correlate poorly with mixed venous pH and pCO_2.[28] When these measurements are not available, subsequent doses of sodium bicarbonate (0.5 mEq/kg) may be given every 10 minutes by slow (1–2 minutes) infusion if the cardiac arrest continues.

Precautions: Excessive sodium bicarbonate may result in metabolic alkalosis, which has the following detrimental effects: 1) displacement of the oxyhemoglobin dissociation curve to the left with impaired tissue oxygen delivery;[29] 2) acute shift of potassium intracellularly with a lowering of serum potassium concentration; 3) a decreased plasma ionized calcium concentration by enhancing its binding to serum proteins, and 4) decreased fibrillation threshold.[30] Sodium and water overload are also potential problems since 1 mEq of sodium is delivered with each milliequivalent of bicarbonate. The standard 8.4% solution of sodium bicarbonate is very hyperosmolar (2,000 mOsm/L) compared to plasma (280 mOsm/L). Repeated doses can therefore result in symptomatic hypernatremia and hyperosmolality.[31] In premature infants this hyperosmolarity has been associated with central nervous system hemorrhage.

Carbon dioxide production is transiently enhanced following sodium bicarbonate administration. This newly formed carbon dioxide can cross the blood–brain barrier and cell membranes much more rapidly than HCO_3^- and cause paradoxical cerebrospinal fluid and intracellular acidosis.[21,24] This is particularly problematic in patients in whom metabolic acidosis has been longstanding (e.g., diabetic ketoacidosis).

Catecholamines are inactivated by, and calcium salts will precipitate in, bicarbonate solutions. It is important to flush the IV before and after infusions of sodium bicarbonate. Since sodium bicarbonate is hyperosmolar, it is sclerosing to small veins and produces a chemical burn if extravasated into the subcutaneous tissues. For this reason it cannot be given into the tracheobronchial tree.

Available Preparations: Sodium bicarbonate is available in prefilled syringes:

50 ml of 8.4% solution (1 mEq/mL)
10 ml of 8.4% solution (1 mEq/mL)
10 ml of 4.2% solution (0.5 mEq/mL) — for infants < 3 months old.

D. Atropine

1. Therapeutic Considerations

Atropine sulfate is a parasympatholytic drug that accelerates sinus or atrial pacemakers as well as atrioventricular conduction.

2. Indications

Atropine is used to treat bradycardia when accompanied by poor perfusion or hypotension, to diminish the vagally mediated bradycardia accompanying intubation attempts, and in the uncommon event of symptomatic bradycardia with atrioventricular block. It may also be useful in asystole. In the small infant (< 6 months), cardiac output is rate dependent; bradycardia (heart rate < 80 beats/min) in a distressed infant needs to be treated, even if blood pressure is normal. In an emergency, bradycardia most often results from hypoxemia. Therefore, treatment should *initially* be directed at ventilation and oxygenation rather than the administration of atropine.

3. Dose

It is important to give a vagolytic dose of atropine. The recommended dose is 0.02 mg/kg with a minimum dose of 0.1 mg and a maximum of 1.0 mg. This may be repeated at 5-minute intervals to a maximum dose of 1.0 mg in a child and 2.0 mg in an adolescent. Atropine may be given via the endotracheal tube in the same dose used intravenously and via the intraosseous route.

4. Precautions

Tachycardia may follow the administration of atropine, but this is generally well tolerated in the pediatric patient. Low doses of atropine may be accompanied by a paradoxical bradycardia in infants; therefore, a minimum dose of 0.1 mg should be used. When used to block vagal-induced bradycardia during intubation, it is important to recognize that atropine may also mask hypoxemia-induced bradycardia.

5. Available Preparations

Prefilled syringes: 10-mL (0.1 mg/mL)
                                5 mL (0.1 mg/mL)
Vial: 1 mL (1 mg/mL)

E. Glucose

1. Therapeutic Considerations

Glucose is an important agent in the resuscitation of infants and children. Small infants and chronically ill children have limited glycogen stores that are rapidly depleted with stress, and the resultant hypoglycemia may clinically mimic hypoxemia (poor perfusion, diaphoresis, tachycardia, and hypotension). Glucose is the major metabolic substrate of the neonatal myocardium, and vigorous myocardial contraction may not be possible in the face of hypoglycemia.

2. Indications

During cardiac resuscitation of an infant or child, a rapid bedside glucose test should be obtained and glucose administered if hypoglycemia is present. It may also be indicated in infants and children who fail to respond to the usual resuscitation measures.

3. Dose

Glucose should be administered in a dose of 0.5–1.0 g/kg IV. This should be delivered in a solution of $D_{25}W$ or less. Since glucose is supplied as $D_{50}W$, it must be diluted 1:1

with sterile water. The administered dose of $D_{25}W$ is 2–4 mL/kg. A $D_{10}W$ solution is prepared by diluting the $D_{50}W$ 1:4 with sterile water.

4. Precautions

Even $D_{25}W$ is very hyperosmolar and may be sclerosing to peripheral veins. In addition, repeated administration may result in a hyperosmolar state, which has been associated with intraventricular hemorrhage in the premature infant.

5. Available Preparations

Glucose is available in vials and prefilled syringes containing 50 mL of $D_{50}W$ (0.5 g/mL).

F. Calcium Chloride

1. Therapeutic Considerations

The administration of calcium to treat cardiac arrest was initially extrapolated from the experience of cardiovascular surgeons. In post-bypass patients, calcium administration is associated with a positive inotropic effect.[32] Recent studies have pointed out, however, that calcium entry into the cell cytoplasm is the final common pathway of cell death.[33] It has been suggested that calcium administration may be injurious,[34] and this is supported by the salutary effects of calcium channel blockers in myocardial preservation during cardiopulmonary bypass.[35]

Calcium is essential to the process of excitation–contraction coupling. When cardiac muscle cells are excited, calcium enters the cytoplasm and induces the coupling of actin and myosin. This event is terminated by an active pumping of calcium out of the cytoplasm. In the presence of myocardial ischemia, this pumping mechanism may be compromised by insufficient energy, and calcium may accumulate in the cytoplasm, with toxic consequences.

2. Indications

Calcium has previously been recommended for the treatment of electromechanical dissociation and ventricular asystole.[36] There is no evidence to support its use in asystole, and its value in electromechanical dissociation is questionable.[37] Evidence also suggests that an adrenergic drug such as methoxamine is much more effective in the therapy for electromechanical dissociation than is calcium.[13] Calcium is therefore no longer recommended for either asystole or electromechanical dissociation.[38]

Calcium is indicated when hypocalcemia has been documented or is suspected and should be considered for the treatment of hyperkalemia, which can occur in diseases such as renal failure or following an accidental potassium overdose.[39] Calcium is also indicated in the treatment of hypermagnesemia and calcium channel blocker overdose.

3. Dose

Calcium is available in three different salts. Calcium chloride is the only form that should be considered in resuscitation since it directly delivers ionized calcium, whereas the gluconate and gluceptate salts must be hepatically metabolized to release ionized calcium.[40]

There is little information on the optimal dose of calcium in resuscitation; a recommended dose of 5–7 mg/kg of ionized calcium is based on its safe use in anesthetized patients.[41,42] Calcium chloride is a 10% solution (100 mg/mL of the calcium salt) that contains 1.36 mEq of ionized (elemental) calcium per milliliter (27.2 mg ionized calcium/mL). Therefore, 0.2–0.25 mL/kg of calcium chloride will deliver 5–7 mg/kg of elemental calcium (20–25 mg/kg of calcium salt). Since repeated doses of calcium increase the risk of morbidity, it is recommended that the initial dose may be repeated only one time in 10 minutes and that further doses be based on *measured* calcium deficiency.

4. Precautions

Rapid calcium administration may induce significant bradycardia, and in patients on digoxin, calcium administration may precipitate severe arrhythmias, including sinus arrest. Calcium forms an insoluble precipitate in the presence of sodium bicarbonate. It is sclerosing to peripheral veins, and if the bolus infiltrates, it can produce a severe chemical burn.

5. Available Preparations

Prefilled syringes: 10 mL calcium chloride, 10%
(100 mg/mL = 27.2 mg/mL
elemental calcium)

G. Lidocaine

1. Therapeutic Considerations

Ventricular fibrillation is seen in less than 10% of pediatric cardiac arrests; the most prevalent rhythm disturbances are asystole or bradyarrhythmias.[15] When ventricular fibrillation is present in a child, one should look for a metabolic etiology, such as abnormalities in calcium, potassium, and blood glucose, as well as hypothermia and drug-related causes (particularly tricyclic antidepressant overdose).

Lidocaine has a long history of successful use in ventricular fibrillation and ventricular tachycardia.[43] It suppresses discharge from ectopic foci, increases the fibrillation threshold, and inhibits the formation of reentrant circuits that can lead to ventricular tachycardia or fibrillation. In clinically used doses, lidocaine has no effect on myocardial contractile state, arterial blood pressure, or atrioventricular and intraventricular conduction.

2. Indications

Lidocaine should be administered to the child with ventricular tachycardia or ventricular fibrillation or to the hemodynamically unstable child with ventricular couplets. Its use in a hemodynamically stable child with frequent PVC's is controversial, but probably unnecessary. A constant infusion should be used in ventricular tachycardia or ventricular fibrillation that reverts after a lidocaine bolus.

3. Dose

The recommended dose is 1 mg/kg infused intravenously or via an intraosseous or ET tube route. In pediatric patients this is often sufficient to normalize ventricular arrhythmias or maintain an electrically converted rhythm. Another dose can be given in 10–15 minutes, but if this is required, a continuous infusion should be started. The infusion should contain 120 mg of lidocaine in 100 mL of D_5W, given at a rate of 20–50 µg/kg/min (1–2.5 mL/kg/hr). To assure adequate plasma concentrations, the patient should receive a 1-mg/kg bolus of lidocaine when beginning the infusion. In the presence of shock or known liver disease, the infusion should be started at 1 mL/kg/hr (20 µg/kg/min) to prevent toxicity from impaired lidocaine clearance.

4. Precautions

Excessive doses of lidocaine may produce myocardial and circulatory depression and central nervous system symptoms, including drowsiness, disorientation, muscle twitching, and focal or generalized seizures. Treatment consists of terminating the lidocaine infusion and administering diazepam or phenobarbital if seizures are present.

5. Available Preparations

Prefilled syringes: 5 mL: 100 mg/5 mL (2%)
10 mg/mL (1%)
Vials: 40 mg/mL (4%)

H. Bretylium Tosylate

1. Therapeutic Considerations

Bretylium is an antiarrhythmic agent with complex pharmacology.[44] It appears to have biphasic effects in the intact circulation: There is an initial transient increase in blood pressure and heart rate, followed several minutes later by a decrease in both, while cardiac output remains unchanged. The initial effects are probably mediated by catecholamine release.

2. Indications

There is currently no published information on the use of bretylium in pediatric patients. Studies in adults suggest that bretylium is very effective in making the fibrillating heart susceptible to electrical defibrillation.[45,46] The benefits of bretylium in adults suggest that it would also be useful in children in the treatment of ventricular fibrillation and tachycardia that is resistant to defibriliation (or cardioversion) and lidocaine.

3. Dose

The recommended dose is 5 mg/kg given by rapid intravenous infusion followed by another attempt at electrical defibrillation. If ventricular fibrillation persists, the dose can be increased to 10 mg/kg and the countershock repeated.

Bretylium may also be helpful in refractory or recurrent ventricular tachycardia. It should be administered in a dose of 5 mg/kg over 8–10 minutes since, in the conscious patient, nausea and vomiting may follow more rapid administration. If necessary, this dose may be repeated in 20 minutes.

4. Precautions

Bretylium may induce nausea, vomiting, hypotension (which usually responds to head down positioning and fluid administration), and transient hypertension. Its use in the digitalized patient is controversial since it may potentially worsen the arrhythmia.

5. Available Preparations

Bretylium is available in a 10-mL vial containing 500 mg (50 mg/mL).

IV. Medications for Postresuscitation Stabilization

The following medications are used to help stabilize, in the postresuscitation phase, a child in whom blood pressure or perfusion remains unstable. These medications should not be mixed with sodium bicarbonate or other alkaline solutions that will inactivate them.

A. Isoproterenol

1. Therapeutic Considerations

Isoproterenol is a pure beta-adrenergic agonist and therefore produces an increase in heart rate, conduction velocity, and cardiac contractility. Peripherally, isoproterenol produces vasodilation that is especially prominent in the skeletal muscle vascular bed since this bed contains the most extensive beta-adrenergic innervation. Isoproterenol infusions produce tachycardia and an increase in pulse pressure, characterized by a fall in diastolic pressure and a rise in systolic pressure. Cardiac output increases if circulating blood volume is adequate.[47]

2. Indications

Isoproterenol is indicated for the treatment of hemodynamically significant bradycardia due to heart block and resistant to atropine, or recurring shortly after an atropine dose. In small infants (< 6 months) cardiac output is heart-rate dependent since stroke volume is fairly fixed. Isoproterenol may be used to increase heart rate (if it is < 80 per minute) in the infant with poor perfusion, even if the measured blood pressure is normal. Epinephrine infusion, however, is preferable in this setting since it does not cause as large a fall in diastolic blood pressure (see "Precautions," below).

3. Dose

Isoproterenol has a very short half-life (1.5 minutes) following IV infusion[11] and must be administered by a constant infusion pump rather than in bolus form. The infusion is prepared by placing 0.6 mg (3 mL) of isoproterenol into 100 mL of an appropriate diluent (see "Drug Administration"), which results in a final concentration of 6 µg/mL. Infusion rates of 1 mL/kg/hr will deliver 0.1 µg/kg/min. This is a reasonable starting dose, although infusion rates up to 1.0 µg/kg/min may be needed. The infusion rate should be increased every 5 minutes until an effect is seen. It can then be adjusted to the patient's clinical response, with tachycardia acting as the major limiting factor. Another format for preparing infusions is given in Table 5.1.

4. Precautions

The major action of catecholamines useful in CPR is through an alpha-adrenergic effect that improves coronary perfusion by increasing blood pressure.[12-14] Isoproterenol potentially compromises coronary perfusion since it has no alpha-adrenergic effects and decreases diastolic blood pressure. Experimental studies in adults confirm this detrimental effect.[47] Furthermore, isoproterenol increases myocardial oxygen demand by increasing myocardial contractility and heart rate. The latter causes a further diminution in coronary perfusion by decreasing diastolic filling time. Therefore, isoproterenol should be used only for the treatment of bradycardia, and the infusion should not be advanced beyond that needed to increase the heart rate.

5. Available Preparations

Vials: 5 mL (0.2 mg/mL)

B. Dopamine

1. Therapeutic Considerations

Dopamine is an endogenous catecholamine with complex cardiovascular effects.[11] In low doses dopamine produces little direct cardiac action, but by acting at specific dopamine receptors, it produces vasodilation and, thus, increased blood flow in the renal and splanchnic vascular beds.[48] As the infusion rate of dopamine is increased, it produces both direct stimulation of the cardiac beta-adrenergic receptors and indirect stimulation through the release of norepinephrine stored in cardiac sympathetic nerves.[49,50] If these stores are depleted, dopamine has a diminished inotropic effect. Clinically, a diminished inotropic effect has been seen in patients with chronic congestive heart failure[51] with depleted cardiac norepinephrine stores and in young pediatric patients in whom sympathetic innervation of the ventricular myocardium may be incomplete.[52]

In the peripheral vascular bed, dopamine also has both direct and indirect actions at the alpha- and beta-adrenergic receptors. In low doses the prominent effect is vasodilation;[49] as the dose is increased, alpha-adrenergic vasoconstriction occurs. Clinically, infusion rates of dopamine between 5 and 10 μg/kg/min are associated with increased contractility, often without prominent effects on heart rate and blood pressure.[53] As the infusion rate is increased from 10 to 20 μg/kg/min, blood pressure is progressively increased due to vasoconstriction, and significant tachycardia may occur. It is important to recognize that a patient may not respond in a predictable manner to dopamine infusion because of variability in the patient's own endogenous catecholamine response and in releasable stores of norepinephrine.

2. Indications

Dopamine is indicated in the treatment of hypotension and/or poor peripheral perfusion in the pediatric patient in whom a stable rhythm is present or has been restored. Low doses (1–5 μg/kg/min) enhance renal and splanchnic blood flow.

3. Dose

Dopamine has a short plasma half-life and must be delivered by a constant infusion pump. Infusions can be prepared according to Table 5.1. Another method is to add 60 mg of dopamine into 100 mL of diluent, resulting in a final concentration of 600 μg/mL. Infusions of 1 mL/kg/hr of this mixture deliver 10 μg/kg/min, a reasonable starting dose for the child with shock. The infusion can then be adjusted as indicated by improvement in the patient's per-

Table 5.1. Preparation of Catecholamine Infusions in Infants and Children*

Isoproterenol Epinephrine	0.6 × body weight (in kg) is the mg dose added to make 100 mL	Then 1 mL/hr delivers 0.1 μg/kg/min
Dopamine Dobutamine	6 × body weight (in kg) is the mg dose added to make 100 mL	Then 1 mL/hr delivers 1 μg/kg/min

* This is a starting dose only; subsequently, concentration can be adjusted to fluid tolerance.

    According to the formulas given above, the amount of drug needed to make 100 mL of fluid to deliver the desired dose at the slow infusion rate of 1 mL/hr may necessitate a high volume of medication. If the volume of medication needed is unusually large (usually a problem only with isoproterenol), it is possible to deplete the available drug supply. To reduce the volume of drug needed, decrease the amount mixed by a factor of 10 and increase the hourly infusion rate by a factor of 10. For example, according to the formula above, a 20-kg child would require 12.0 mg (20 × 0.6) or 60 mL (0.2 mg/mL) of isoproterenol. Instead, use 1.2 mg (6 mL) and infuse the final solution at 10 mL/hr (instead of 1 mL/hr).

fusion or blood pressure. Infusion rates above 20 μg/kg/min produce predominant vasoconstrictive effects without any further inotropic effect and should be used with caution. If further inotropic effect is needed, epinephrine, with its alpha- and beta-adrenergic effects, is preferable to infusion of dopamine in excess of 20 μg/kg/min.

4. Precautions

Dopamine may produce tachycardia (which increases myocardial oxygen demand), excessive increases in blood pressure, and arrhythmias, including premature ventricular contractions, supraventricular tachycardia, and ventricular tachycardia.[54] Due to its peripheral vasoconstrictive effects, high infusion rates of dopamine may produce extremity ischemia in the child with shock.

Dopamine infusions should be given into a central vein if possible. A large-bore peripheral IV may be a suitable alternative. Extravasation of the infusion can result in local chemical burns. Dopamine, like other catecholamines, should not be mixed with sodium bicarbonate or other alkaline solutions that will inactivate them.

5. Available Preparations

Vials: 5 mL (40 mg/mL)

C. Dobutamine

1. Therapeutic Considerations

Dobutamine is a synthetic catecholamine possessing relatively selective action at beta₁-adrenergic receptors, resulting in increased cardiac contractility and heart rate with little net effect on peripheral vascular tone.[11,55] Unlike dopamine, dobutamine is a direct-acting catecholamine whose action does not depend on the presence of releasable stores of norepinephrine and it has no selective effect on renal blood flow. There is little published experience with dobutamine in pediatric patients. In children with cardiogenic shock, dobutamine increases cardiac output and decreases pulmonary wedge (occlusive) pressure and systemic vascular resistance.[56,57] It appears to be less effective in septic shock and in infants (< 12 months).[57]

2. Indications

Dobutamine is indicated for the treatment of hypotension and/or poor perfusion in the postresuscitation phase. Although comparative clinical studies are lacking, it has no clear advantages over dopamine, and in the hypotensive patient may not increase blood pressure as effectively as dopamine.

3. Dose

Like other catecholamines, dobutamine has a short plasma half-life and must be infused by a constant infusion pump. Infusions can be prepared according to Table 5.1. Another method is to add 60 mg of dobutamine into

100 mL of diluent, giving a final concentration of 600 μg/mL. Infusions of this solution are then begun at 0.5–1 mL/kg/hr, which delivers 5–10 μg/kg/min. The infusion rate should be adjusted as needed to stabilize the patient's blood pressure and perfusion; infusion rates over 20 μg/kg/min are usually not required.

4. Precautions

Dobutamine may produce tachycardia and/or tachyarrhythmias. Nausea, vomiting, hypertension, and hypotension are less frequent side effects. Like other catecholamines, dobutamine is inactivated in alkaline solutions.

5. Available Preparations

Vials: 10 mL (25 mg/mL).

D. Epinephrine Infusion

1. Therapeutic Considerations

The actions of epinephrine have been reviewed previously. It is a potent direct-acting catecholamine; i.e., it acts directly on the adrenergic receptors rather than through a release of stored norepinephrine. Epinephrine has dose-related actions in which low-dose infusions (< 0.3 μg/kg/min) are primarily associated with beta-adrenergic effects,[49] including an increase in myocardial contractility, heart rate, and pulse pressure, with an increase in systolic, but a fall in diastolic, pressure. As the infusion is increased beyond 0.3 μg/kg/min, increasing alpha-adrenergic action occurs, characterized by increases in both systolic and diastolic blood pressure.

2. Indications

The indications for epinephrine infusion are hypotension, poor perfusion following the restoration of a stable rhythm, and hemodynamically significant bradycardia. Epinephrine is preferred for the patient who may have depleted myocardial norepinephrine stores, such as the young infant or the chronically stressed patient.

3. Dose

Epinephrine infusions should be delivered through either a well-secured peripheral IV or, preferably, a central line. The infusion can be prepared according to Table 5.1. Another method is to add 0.6 mg of epinephrine into 100 mL of diluent, resulting in a final concentration of 6 μg/mL. Infusion rates of 1 mL/kg/hr of this mixture will deliver 0.1 μg/kg/min, which is a reasonable starting dose. Since epinephrine has a short half-life (approximately 2 minutes), the infusion rate should be adjusted every 5 minutes until the desired clinical effect is achieved. Dosages of up to approximately 1.0 μg/kg/min may be used with caution.

4. Precautions

Epinephrine can produce significant supraventricular or ventricular tachycardia and ventricular ectopy. High-dose

Table 5.2. Drugs Used in Pediatric Cardiopulmonary Resuscitation and Postresuscitation Stablization

Drug	Dose	How Supplied*	Remarks
Epinephrine hydrochloride	0.01 mg/kg 0.1 mL/kg	1:10,000 (0.1 mg/mL)	Most useful drug in cardiac arrest; 1:1,000 must be diluted.
Sodium bicarbonate	1 mEq/kg 1 mL/kg	1 mEq/mL (8.4% soln)	Infuse slowly and *only* when ventilation is adequate.
Atropine sulfate	0.02 mg/kg 0.2 mL/kg	0.1 mg/mL	Minimum dose of 0.1 mg (1 mL); use for bradycardia after assessing ventilation. Maximum dose: infants and children = 1.0 mg; adolescents = 2.0 mg
Calcium chloride	20 mg/kg (0.2 mL/kg)	100 mg/mL (10% soln)	Use only for hypocalcemia, calcium blocker overdose, hyperkalemia or hypermagnesemia; give slowly.
Glucose	0.5–1.0 g/kg	0.5 g/mL D$_{50}$W	Dilute 1:1 with water (D$_{25}$W): dose is then 2–4 mL/kg.
Lidocaine hydrochloride	1 mg/kg	10 mg/mL (1%) 20 mg/mL (2%)	Used for ventricular arrhythmias only.
Bretylium tosylate	5 mg/kg	50 mg/mL	Use if lidocaine is not effective; repeat dose with 10 mg/kg if first dose not effective.
Infusions			
Epinephrine infusion	0.1–1.0 μg/ kg/min	1 mg/mL 1:1,000	Titrate infusion to desired hemodynamic effect.
Dopamine hydrochloride infusion	2–20 μg/kg/ min	40 mg/mL	Titrate to desired hemodynamic response.
Dobutamine infusion	5–20 μg/kg/ min	250 mg/vial lyophilized	Titrate to desired hemodynamic response; may cause vasodilation.
Isoproterenol infusion	0.1–1.0 μg/ kg/min	1 mg/5 mL	Titrate to desired hemodynamic effect; vasodilitation.
Lidocaine infusion	20–50 μg/ kg/min	40 mg/mL (4%)	Use lower infusion dose with shock, liver disease.

* For IV push medications, preparation listed is form available in prefilled syringes.

infusions ($> 0.5-0.6$ μg/kg/min) can produce profound vasoconstriction, severe enough to compromise extremity and skin blood flow. Even in lower doses, epinephrine decreases renal blood flow,[58] but improvement in cardiac output in patients with shock improves renal function as assessed by urine output.[59] Infiltration of an epinephrine infusion can cause local ischemia and ulceration of the skin.

5. Available Preparations

Vials (1:1,000): 1 mg/mL. Do not use the prefilled syringes (1:10,000 dilution) for making infusions.

V. Summary

The drug therapies discussed in this chapter are summarized in Table 5.2.

References

1. Rossetti V, Thompson BM, Aprahamian C, et al: Difficulty and delay in intravascular access in pediatric arrests, abstracted. *Ann Emerg Med* 13:406, 1984.
2. Ward JT Jr: Endotracheal drug therapy. *Am J Emerg Med* 1:71, 1983.
3. Roberts JR, Greenberg MI, Knaub MA, et al: Blood levels following intravenous and endotracheal epinephrine administration. *JACEP* 8:53, 1979.
4. Roberts JR, Greenberg MI, Knaub MA, et al: Comparison of the pharmacological effects of epinephrine administered by the intravenous and endotracheal routes. *JACEP* 7:260, 1978.
5. Ralston SH, Voorhees WD, Babbs CF: Intrapulmonary epinephrine during prolonged cardiopulmonary resuscitation: Improved regional blood flow and resuscitation in dogs. *Ann Emerg Med* 13:79, 1984.
6. Hedges JR, Barsan WB, Doan LA, et al: Central versus peripheral intravenous routes in cardiopulmonary resuscitation. *Am J Emerg Med* 2:385, 1984.
7. Dalsey WC, Barsan WG, Joyce SM, et al: Comparison of superior vena caval and inferior vena caval access using a radioisotope technique during normal perfusion and cardiopulmonary resuscitation. *Ann Emerg Med* 13:881, 1984.
8. Berg RA: Emergency infusion of catecholamines into bone marrow. *Am J Dis Child* 138:810, 1984.
9. Thompson BM, Rossetti V, Miller J, et al: Intraosseous administration of sodium bicarbonate: An effective means of pH normalization in the canine model. *Ann Emerg Med* 13:405, 1984.
10. Ditchey RV, Lindenfeld J: Potential adverse effects of volume loading on perfusion of vital organs during closed-chest resuscitation. *Circulation* 69:181, 1984.
11. Zaritsky A, Chernow B: Use of catecholamines in pediatrics. *J Pediatr* 105:341, 1985.
12. Otto CW, Yakaitis RW, Blitt CD: Mechanism of action of epinephrine in resuscitation from asphyxial arrest. *Crit Care Med* 9:321, 1981.
13. Redding JS, Haynes RR, Thomas JD: Drug therapy in resuscitation from electromechanical dissociation. *Crit Care Med* 11:681, 1983.
14. Otto CW: Cardiovascular pharmacology II: The use of cathecholamines, pressor agents, digitalis, and corticosteroids in CPR and emergency cardiac care. *Circulation* 74 (Suppl IV):IV-80, 1986.
15. Friesen RM, Duncan P, Tweed WA, et al: Appraisal of pediatric cardiopulmonary resuscitation. *Can Med Assoc J* 126:1055, 1982.
16. Mitchell JH, Wildenthal K, Johnson RL Jr: The effects of acid–base disturbances on cardiovascular and pulmonary function. *Kidney Int* 1:375, 1972.

17. Chernow B, Holbrook P, D'Angona DS, et al: Epinephrine absorption after intratracheal administration. *Anesth Analg* 63:829, 1984.
18. Roberts JR, Greenberg MI, Knaub MA, et al: Blood levels following intravenous and endotracheal epinephrine administration. *JACEP* 8:53, 1979.
19. Ostrea EM Jr, Odell GB: The influence of bicarbonate administration on blood pH in a "closed system": Clinical implications. *J Pediatr* 80:671, 1972.
20. Rhodes PG, Hall RT, Hellerstein S: The effects of single infusion of hypertonic sodium bicarbonate on body composition in neonates with acidosis. *J Pediatr* 90:789, 1977.
21. Berenyi KJ, Wolk M, Killip T: Cerebrospinal fluid acidosis complicating therapy of experimental cardiopulmonary arrest. *Circulation* 52:319, 1975.
22. Steenbergen C, Deleeuw G, Rich T, Williamson JR: Effects of acidosis and ischemia on contractility and intracellular pH of rat heart. *Circ Res* 41:849, 1977.
23. Clancy RL, Cingolani HE, Taylor RR, Graham TP Jr, Gilmore JP: Influence of sodium bicarbonate on myocardial performance. *Am J Physiol* 212:917, 1967.
24. Arieff AI, Leach W, Park R, Lazarowitz VC: Systemic effects of $NaHCO_3$ in experimental lactic acidosis in dogs. *Am J Physiol* 242:F586, 1982.
25. Eisenberg M, Bergner L, Hallstrom A: Epidemiology of cardiac arrest and resuscitation in children. *Ann Emerg Med* 12:672, 1983.
26. Cohen RD, Simpson BR, Goodwin FJ, et al: The early effects of infusion of sodium bicarbonate and sodium lactate on intracellular hydrogen ion activity in dogs. *Clin Sci* 33:233, 1967.
27. Graf H, Leach W, Arieff AI: Evidence for a detrimental effect of bicarbonate therapy in hypoxic lactic acidosis. *Science* 227:754, 1985.
28. Weil MH, Rackow EC, Trevino R, et al: Difference in acid–base state between venous and arterial blood during cardiopulmonary resuscitation. *N Engl J Med* 315:153, 1986.
29. Bellingham AJ, Detter JC, Lenfant C: Regulatory mechanisms of hemoglobin oxygen affinity in acidosis and alkalosis. *J Clin Invest* 50:700, 1971.
30. Bishop RL, Weisfeldt ML: Sodium bicarbonate administration during cardiac arrest. Effect on arterial pH, PCO_2, and osmolality. *JAMA* 235:506, 1976.
31. Mattar JA, Weil MH, Shubin H, et al: Cardiac arrest in the critically ill. II. Hyperosmolal states following cardiac arrest. *Am J Med* 56:162, 1974.
32. Stulz PM, Scheidegger D, Drop LJ, et al: Ventricular pump performance during hypocalcemia. *J Thorac Cardiovasc Surg* 78:185, 1979.
33. Katz AM, Reuter H: Cellular calcium and cardiac cell death. *Am J Cardiol* 44:188, 1979.
34. Dembo DH: Calcium in advanced life support. *Crit Care Med* 9:358, 1981.
35. Clark RE, Christlieb IY, Ferguson TB, Marbarger JP, et al: The first American trial of nifedipine in cardioplegia. A report of the first 12 month experience. *J Thorac Cardiovasc Surg* 82:848, 1981.
36. Standards and guidelines for cardiopulmonary resuscitation (CPR) and emergency cardiac care (ECC). *JAMA* 244:453, 1980.
37. Steuven HA, Thompson B, Aprahamian C, et al: The effectiveness of calcium chloride in refractory electromechanical dissocation. *Ann Emerg Med* 14:626, 1985.
38. Standards and guidelines for cardiopulmonary resuscitation (CPR) and emergency cardiac care (ECC). *JAMA* 255:2933, 1986.
39. Oh MS, Carroll HJ: Electrolyte disorders, in Chernow B, Lake CR, (eds): *The Pharmacologic Approach to the Critically Ill Patient.* Baltimore, Williams and Wilkins, 1983, p. 715.
40. White RD, Goldsmith RS, Rodriguez R, et al: Plasma ionic calcium levels following injection of chloride, gluconate, and gluceptate salts of calcium. *J Thorac Cardiovasc Surg* 71:609, 1976.
41. Lappas DG, Drop LJ, Buckley MJ, et al: Hemodynamic response to calcium chloride during coronary artery surgery. *Surg Forum* 26:234, 1975.
42. Denlinger JK, Kaplan JA, Lecky JH, et al: Cardiovascular responses to calcium administered to man during halothane anesthesia. *Anesthesiology* 42:390, 1975.
43. Collinsworth KA, Kalman SM, Harrison DC: The clinical pharmacology of lidocaine as an anti-arrhythmic drug. *Circulation* 50:1217, 1975.

44. Dronen SC: Antifibrillatory drugs: The case for bretylium tosylate. *Ann Emerg Med* 13(Part 2):805, 1984.
45. Holder DA, Sniderman AD, Fraser G, et al: Experience with bretylium tosylate by a hospital cardiac arrest team. *Circulation* 55:541, 1977.
46. Stang JM, Washington SE, Barnes SA, et al: Treatment of pre-hospital refractory ventricular fibrillation with bretylium tosylate. *Ann Emerg Med* 13:234, 1984.
47. Mueller H, Ayres SM, Gregory JJ, et al: Hemodynamics, coronary blood flow and myocardial metabolism in coronary shock: Response to l-norepinephrine and isoproterenol. *J Clin Invest* 49:1885, 1977.
48. Goldberg LI, Volkman PH, Kohli JD: A comparison of the vascular dopamine receptor with other dopamine receptors. *Ann Rev Pharmacol Toxicol* 18:57, 1978.
49. Goldberg LI, Hsieh YY, Resnekov L: Newer catecholamines for treatment of heart failure and shock: An update on dopamine and a first look at dobutamine. *Prog Cardiovasc Dis* 19:327, 1977.
50. Farmer JB: Indirect sympathomimetic action of dopamine. *J Pharm Pharmacol* 18:261, 1966.
51. Leier CV, Heban PT, Huss P, et al: Comparative systemic and regional hemodynamic effects of dopamine and dobutamine in patients with cardiomyopathic heart failure. *Circulation* 58:466, 1978.
52. Driscoll DJ, Gillette PC, Ezrailson EG, et al: Inotropic response of the neonatal canine myocardium to dopamine. *Pediatr Res* 12:42, 1978.
53. Goldberg LI: Dopamine — Clinical use of an endogenous catecholamine. *New Engl J Med* 291:707, 1974.
54. Guller B, Fields AI, Coleman MG, et al: Changes in cardiac rhythm in children treated with dopamine. *Crit Care Med* 6:151, 1978.
55. Leier CV, Unverferth DV: Drugs five years later: Dobutamine. *Ann Intern Med* 99:490, 1983.
56. Schranz D, Stopfkuchen H, Jungst BK, et al: Hemodynamic effects of dobutamine in children with cardiovascular failure. *Eur J Pediatr* 139:4, 1982.
57. Perkin RM, Levin DL, Webb R, et al: Dobutamine: A hemodynamic evaluation in children with shock. *J Pediatr* 100:977, 1982.
58. Gombos EA, Hulet WH, Bopp P, et al: Reactivity of renal and systemic circulations to vasoconstrictor agents in normotensive and hypertensive subjects. *J Clin Invest* 41:203, 1962.
59. Coffin LH Jr, Ankeney JL, Beheler EM: Experimental study and clinical use of epinephrine for treatment of low cardiac output syndrome. *Circulation* 33 (Suppl I):I-78, 1966.
60. Ralston SH, Tacker WA, Showen L, Babbs CF: Endotracheal versus intravenous epinephrine during electromechanical dissociation with CPR in dogs. *Ann Emerg Med* 14:1044, 1985.
61. Brown CG, Werman HA: Adrenergic agonists during cardiopulmonary resuscitation. *Resuscitation* 19:1, 1990.

Cardiac Rhythm Disturbances   Chapter 6

Life-threatening cardiac rhythm disturbances in infants and children are more often the result rather than the cause of acute emergencies. Primary cardiac arrest is infrequent in this age group; more commonly, cardiac arrest is the end result of a long period of hypoxemia and acidosis secondary to respiratory insufficiency. During an acute emergency in the pediatric age group, therefore, attention must first be directed toward maintaining a patent airway, good ventilation, adequate oxygenation, and circulatory stabilization. This chapter is limited to a discussion of the arrhythmias most commonly associated with emergency situations requiring cardiopulmonary resuscitation and is not intended as a complete discussion of cardiac arrhythmias in pediatrics.

I. The Normal Electrocardiogram

The surface electrocardiogram (ECG) is a graphic representation of the sequence of myocardial depolarization, with each normal cardiac cycle consisting of a P, a QRS, and a T wave (Figure 6.1). Electrical depolarization begins in the sinoatrial node, located at the junction of the superior vena cava and right atrium, and advances via atrial tissue and the internodal pathways to the atrioventricular node (AV), where it is temporarily slowed. It then progresses via the bundle of His and its divisions to depolarize the endocardium of both ventricles (Figure 6.2). The first wave (P) represents depolarization of both atria. The AV nodal delay and subsequent spread via the bundle of His is included in the P–R interval, while the QRS represents depolarization of the ventricular myocardium. Ventricular repolarization is seen on the surface ECG as the S–T segment and the T wave (Figure 6.3).

The normal heart rate in children is related to age and is influenced by the level of activity and the presence of pathologic conditions such as fever, blood loss, etc. Table 6.1 is a composite of several studies[1-4] and shows the wide variation in the normal rate as well as the gradual decline with age. It should be appreciated that a febrile infant with a normal cardiovascular state can achieve heart rates close to 200 beats/min. In the sick infant, the differentiation of sinus tachycardia from paroxysmal supraventricular tachycardia as a cause of vascular collapse can be problematic and is discussed below.

II. Monitoring the Electrocardiogram

The electrocardiogram should be continuously monitored in any child who has sustained a cardiopulmonary arrest and in any child at risk of an arrest. One limitation of electrocardiographic monitoring is that it gives no information about the effectiveness of myocardial contractility or the adequacy of tissue perfusion. Management decisions must therefore always be based on the clinical evaluation of the patient correlated with information derived from the electrocardiogram.

A. Hardware

A cardiac monitor usually consists of a screen on which the electrocardiogram may be viewed, a heart rate tachometer that automatically calculates the heart rate from the R–R interval, and often, a direct writer that provides a hard copy of the tracing. Some monitors also have memory so that rhythm disturbances can be stored for later recall and analysis. An ECG machine may be

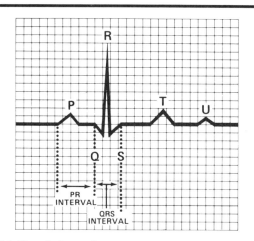

Figure 6.1. The electrocardiogram.

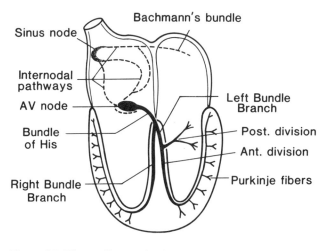

Figure 6.2. The cardiac conduction system.

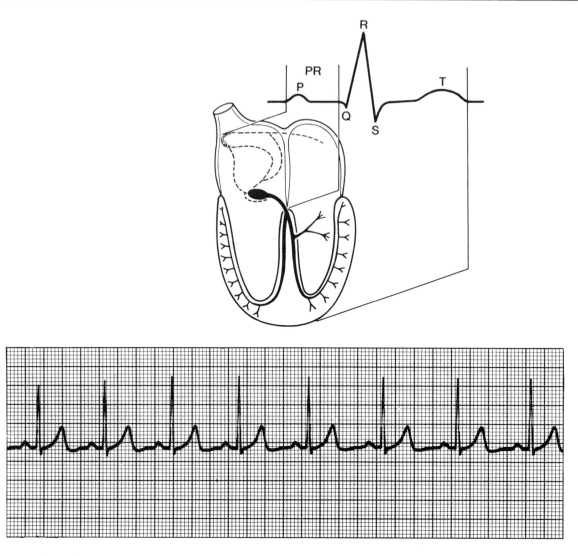

Figure 6.3. The relationship of the electrocardiogram to the anatomy of the conduction system.

used as a monitor, but one of its disadvantages is the waste of a great deal of recording paper.

A cardiac monitor is connected to the patient via three color-coded cables attached to disposable adhesive monitoring pads or via metal electrodes. The latter are usually attached to the extremities while the former may be attached either to the chest or the extremities. Both are available in the small sizes convenient for pediatric patients. Disposable adhesive disc electrodes should be attached in locations 1) that record a rhythm strip of good quality with visible P waves, 2) in which the R wave, but not the T wave, triggers the tachometer, and 3) that are free of artifact. As much of the chest as possible should be left free for chest compressions, should they become necessary, and for auscultation of the heart and lungs. Electrodes are best placed on the shoulders or the lateral chest surfaces, with the ground electrode on the abdomen or thigh (Figure 6.4).

B. Artifacts

Everyone using a monitoring system must be familiar with potential artifacts. Three common artifacts are as follows:

1. A straight line, resembling asystole, or a wavy line, resembling coarse fibrillation, can be caused by a loose wire or monitoring electrode.
2. If the T wave is tall, it can be mistaken by the tachometer as an R wave and result in a heart rate reading twice the actual rate ("double counting").
3. Lead placement that is perpendicular to the P wave axis may make it appear as if P waves are absent.

These and other potential artifacts emphasize the importance of clinical assessment and correlation before therapeutic decisions are made.

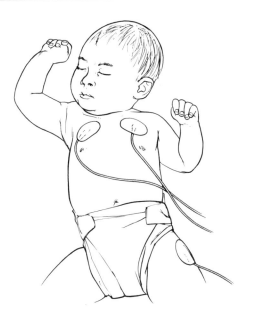

Figure 6.4. Placement of electrodes for electrocardiographic monitoriing.

III. Abnormal Rhythms

A. Principles of Therapy

In children, a rhythm disturbance should be treated as an emergency only if:

- it compromises the cardiac output or
- it has the potential for degenerating into a lethal rhythm.

Cardiac output is the product of stroke volume (SV) and heart rate (HR). Therefore, *very rapid rates*, which compromise diastolic filling and preclude adequate stroke volume, and *very slow rates* may both adversely influence the cardiac output.

For therapeutic purposes, in the setting of cardiopulmonary resuscitation, it is useful to classify the arrhythmias into:

- fast heart rates: the tachyarrhythmias
- slow heart rates: the bradyarrhythmias
- disorganized or collapse rhythms

Other rhythm disturbances, such as premature atrial, junctional, or ventricular beats, may need further cardiac evaluation but usually do not require emergency treatment in children and are not common causes or consequences of cardiopulmonary arrest.

When *rapid rates* produce cardiovascular instability, they should be treated by the most rapid and effective method — synchronized cardioversion. (In the nonemergency situation there are, of course, other methods of management, but a discussion of these is beyond the purpose of this chapter.)

The *slow* rhythms associated with an acute cardiopulmonary emergency in children usually result from atrioventricular block or suppression of normal impulse generation caused by a combination of acidosis and hypoxemia. Initial therapy consists of proper ventilation and oxygenation; if needed, medications, e.g., atropine and sympathomimetics, may be used.

B. The Tachyarrhythmias

1. Sinus Tachycardia (ST)

This is due to a rate of sinus node discharge higher than normal for age (see Table 6.1). Etiology includes anxiety, fever, pain, blood loss, and any other insult in which an increased cardiac output is needed.

Table 6.1. Heart Rates in Normal Children[1–4]

Age	Range	Mean
Newborn to 3 mo	85–205	140
3 mo to 2 yr	100–190	130
2 yr to 10 yr	60–140	80
> 10 yr	60–100	75

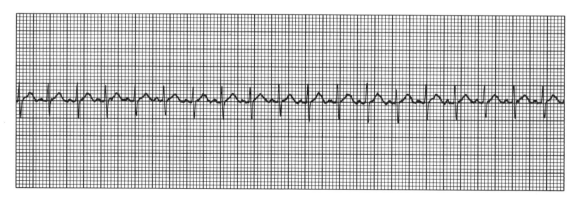

Figure 6.5. Sinus tachycardia (180 beat/min) in a febrile 3-year-old child.

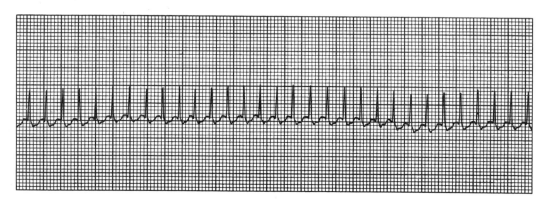

Figure 6.6. Supraventricular tachycardia in an infant. The heart rate is 320 beats/min.

Figure 6.7. Ventricular tachycardia. The rhythm is regular at a rate of 158 beats/min. The QRS is wide. No evidence of atrial depolarization is seen.

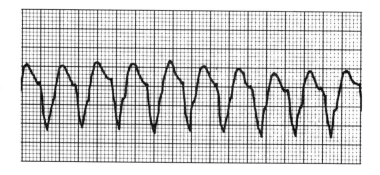

ECG Criteria: (See Figure 6.5.) a) Rate greater than normal for age, b) regular rhythm with normal P, QRS, T sequence.

Therapy: Therapy is directed at the underlying cause.

2. Supraventricular Tachycardia (SVT)

This is a rapid regular rhythm, usually caused by a reentry mechanism, which originates above the bifurcation of the bundle of His. It is often paroxysmal and, though usually well tolerated in older children, can cause cardiovascular collapse, with clinical evidence of shock, in infants.[5,6]

ECG Criteria: (See Figure 6.6.) a) Heart rate varies with age; in infants it may be approximately 240 beats/min but can be as high as 300 beats/min. The rhythm is usually

regular since associated atrioventricular block is rare. b) P waves may not be identifiable at higher rates. c) QRS duration is normal more than 90% of the time;[7] a wide QRS from aberrant conduction is rare in infants and children but, if present, may be difficult to distinguish from ventricular tachycardia. d) S–T and T wave changes consistent with myocardial ischemia may be seen if the tachycardia is of long duration.

In severely ill infants it may be difficult to distinguish sinus tachycardia secondary to an underlying illness (most commonly sepsis or hypovolemia) from SVT on a reentrant basis with secondary shock. The following may be of help in the differentiation:

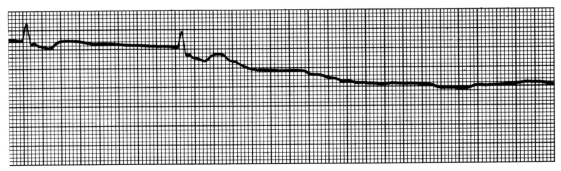

Figure 6.8. Ventricular asystole. Only two QRS complexes are seen, probably representing ventricular escape beats. This is followed by the absence of organized electrical activity.

1. *Heart Rate:* In sinus tachycardia, usually < 200 beats/min. In SVT, more likely > 220 beats/min.
2. *ECG:* P waves may be difficult to see in both at rates > 200 beats/min. In sinus tachycardia the rate may vary from beat to beat. In SVT there is no beat-to-beat variation. Termination of the SVT is abrupt.
3. *Chest X-Ray:* In SVT sufficient to cause cardiovascular instability, heart size may be enlarged. In sinus tachycardia, depending on the cause, it is often normal.

Therapy: a) Synchronized cardioversion [0.5–1.0 J/kg (J=joules, or watt-seconds)] is the treatment of choice for patients with cardiovascular instability. If the SVT persists, the dose is increased to 2.0 J/kg. If conversion still does not occur, consider that the diagnosis may not be correct; the child may have sinus tachycardia. b) In nonemergency situations various techniques and medications are used, but a discussion of these is beyond the scope of this chapter. Caution is advised in using verapamil in infants since cardiovascular collapse has been reported in association with its use.[8,9]

3. Ventricular Tachycardia (VT)

Originating in the ventricles, this arrhythmia is not common in the pediatric age group. Heart rate may vary from close to normal to above 400 beats/min. Slow rates may be well tolerated, but rapid rates compromise cardiac output and may degenerate into ventricular fibrillation. The majority of children with VT have underlying structural heart disease or a prolonged QT interval. Other causes include hypoxia, acidosis, electrolyte imbalance, and insults caused by medications and poisons, especially the tricyclic antidepressants.

ECG Criteria: (See Figure 6.7.) a) Rate is at least 120 beats/min and is regular. b) QRS is wide (> 0.08 seconds). c) P waves are often not seen; when present, they may not be related to QRS (A–V dissociation). At slower rates, atria may be depolarized in a retrograde manner. d) T waves are usually opposite in polarity to the QRS. e) It may be difficult to differentiate SVT with, aberrant conduction from VT; fortunately, aberrant conduction

is present in less than 10% of children with SVT. Wide QRS tachycardia in an infant or child must be considered as ventricular tachycardia until proven otherwise.

Therapy: a) In the presence of cardiovascular instability with clinical evidence of a low cardiac output, use synchronized cardioversion (0.5–1.0 J/kg). b) Lidocaine bolus (1.0 mg/kg) prior to cardioversion results in a higher success rate; infusion therapy with lidocaine 20–50 µg/kg/min will help stabilize the rhythm. c) If cardioversion needs to be repeated, use 2.0 J/kg. d) If lidocaine is unsuccessful, use bretylium (see Chapter 5).

C. The Bradyarrhythmias

Hypoxemia, hypotension, and acidosis interfere with normal function of the sinus and atrioventricular nodes and slow conduction through the normal pathways. Sinus bradycardia, sinus node arrest with a slow junctional or ventricular escape, and various degrees of atrioventricular block are the most common terminal rhythms in children with cardiopulmonary arrest.[10]

ECG Criteria: Rate is slow; P waves may or may not be present, and QRS duration may be normal or prolonged, depending on the pacemaker focus. The relation between P and QRS is often lost. In the context of cardiopulmonary resuscitation, it is not important to diagnose the exact rhythm, but sufficient to identify it as "too slow."

Therapy: Slow rhythms are treated by ensuring good ventilation and oxygenation, chest compressions, atropine, and sympathomimetic medications, especially epinephrine (see Chapter 5).

D. Collapsed or Disorganized Rhythms

1. Asystole

Asystole is clinically diagnosed in a nonbreathing infant or child by the absence of a palpable pulse.

ECG Criteria: (See Figure 6.8.) Straight line on ECG monitor; occasionally P waves are seen. Clinical correlation (absent pulse, absent spontaneous respirations, poor

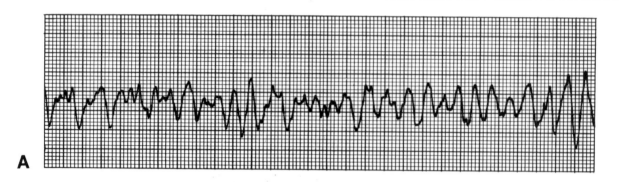

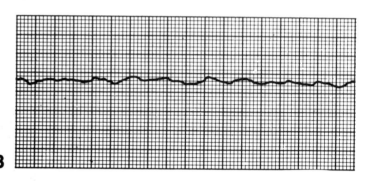

Figure 6.9. Ventricular fibrillation. (A) Coarse VF. Note high-amplitude waveforms which vary in size, shape, and rhythm, representing chaotic ventricular electrical activity. (B) Fine VF. Electrical activity is much reduced.

perfusion) is mandatory since a straight line may also be seen when an ECG monitoring lead is loose.

Therapy: The appropriate steps of ALS for cardiac arrest.

2. Ventricular Fibrillation

Ventricular fibrillation (VF) is a chaotic disorganized series of depolarizations that result in a quivering myocardium without an organized contraction and, therefore, without a detectable pulse. VF is an uncommon terminal event in the pediatric age group (9%)[11] and is especially rare in infants. When an infant or child is found to be without a pulse, therapy should first be directed to achieving adequate ventilation and oxygenation and to maintaining circulation by manual external chest compressions. Defibrillation should be attempted *only* if VF is demonstrated by ECG monitoring.

ECG Criteria: (Figure 6.9.) There are no identifiable P, QRS, or T waves. VF has been classified as coarse or fine by the height of the waves.

Therapy: Cardiopulmonary resuscitation is continued, and, as soon as possible, electrical defibrillation (see below) is attempted.

E. Electromechanical Dissociation

In electromechanical dissociation there is evidence of organized electrical activity on ECG but failure of effective myocardial contractions, as evidenced by the absence of a palpable pulse. The mechanism is not understood. Underlying causes, which must be looked for and cor-

rected if present, include hypoxemia, severe acidosis, tension pneumothorax, and hypovolemia.

IV. Defibrillation and Synchronized Cardioversion[12]

Defibrillation is the untimed (asynchronous) depolarization of a critical mass of myocardial cells that allows a spontaneous organized beat to be initiated. The same principle is used in cardioverting the tachyarrhythmias, but the depolarization used then is timed (synchronous) so as to avoid the vulnerable period of the cardiac cycle.

A. Paddle Size

The ideal paddle size for the pediatric patient is not currently known. The largest electrode size that allows good chest contact over its entire area and good separation between the two electrodes is preferred. Among currently available electrode paddles, the 4.5 cm diameter paddle is adequate for infants; the 8.0 and 13 cm, for older children.

B. Electrode Interface

Since the skin acts as a resistor between the electrode paddles and the heart, a low-impedance interface medium (i.e., electrode gel or cream) is recommended. Sonographic gels are unacceptable since they are poor electrical conductors; saline-soaked pads are also best avoided since their conductivity is variable and they have a tendency to drip, thus potentially producing a short circuit. Alcohol pads are a fire hazard and can produce serious chest burns.

C. Electrode Position

Effective defibrillation depends on an adequate current traversing the heart. The electrode paddles must be placed so that the heart is situated between them. An anterior–posterior arrangement, with one electrode on the anterior chest over the heart and the other on the back, is theoretically superior but impractical during a resuscitation. The standard placement is one paddle on the upper right chest below the clavicle and the other to the left of the left nipple in the anterior axillary line. A mirror image is used in the case of dextrocardia.

D. Energy Dose

The optimal energy dose for the defibrillation of infants and children has not been conclusively established. The controversy over a relation between patient weight and optimal energy dose is recognized. Nevertheless, the available data in the pediatric age group suggest that a dose of 2 J/kg be used initially. If defibrillation is not successful, the dose should be doubled and repeated twice, if necessary. If VF continues, attention should be turned to adequacy of ventilation, oxygenation, and correction of acidosis before another attempt is made. An increase in energy is not required when the rhythm converts and then degenerates back into VF. Either lidocaine or bretylium (see Chapter 5) are used in such instances to raise the fibrillation threshold.

E. Defibrillator Testing

There may be a significant variation between the stored and delivered energy, especially at the very low settings required for infants. All defibrillators should be checked periodically for safety according to standards of the Inter-Society Commission for Heart Disease Resources, and the accuracy of the delivered energy dose should be checked against a 50-ohm resistance. It is important that defibrillators used for infants and children be checked at very low energy doses and that any variations be prominently displayed on the machine.

F. Defibrillation Sequence

If VF is seen on the monitoring system:

1. Continue CPR with as little interruption as possible.
2. Apply conductive medium to appropriately sized paddles.
3. Turn on defibrillator power and be sure that it is not in the synchronous mode.
4. Select the energy dose and charge the capacitor.
5. Stop chest compressions, place paddles in proper position on the chest.
6. Recheck rhythm on monitor.

7. Clear area to make sure that no personnel are in contact with the patient or the bed.
8. Apply firm pressure to the paddles while depressing both discharge buttons simultaneously.
9. Reassess ECG and pulse.
   a. If VF persists, repeat countershock using twice the energy.
   b. If an organized rhythm has been established, check pulse and continue CPR as required.
   c. If VF recurs, immediately repeat countershock using the same dose.

G. Synchronized Cardioversion Sequence

The procedure is the same as that outlined for defibrillation except as follows:

1. If the paddles are not of the monitoring type, the ECG must be connected to the defibrillator.
2. The synchronizer circuit must be activated (a light blinks and a marker is seen on the monitor with each QRS). On some older models, the QRS must be upright for proper activation.
3. The discharge buttons must be pressed and held until the countershock is delivered.

References

1. Alimurung MM, Joseph LG, Nadas AS, et al: The unipolar precordial and extremity electrocardiogram in normal infants and children. *Circulation* 4:420, 1951.
2. Ziegler RF: *Electrocardiographic Studies in Normal Infants and Children.* Springfield, Ill., Charles C. Thomas, 1951.
3. Furman RA, Halloran WR: Electrocardiogram in the first two months of life. *J Pediatr* 39:307, 1951.
4. Tudbury PB, Atkinson DW: Electrocardiograms of 100 normal infants and young children. *J Pediatr* 34:466, 1950.
5. Olley PH: Cardiac arrhythmias, in Keith JD, Rowe RD, Vlad P (eds): *Heart Disease in Infancy and Childhood,* 3 ed. New York, Macmillan Publishing Co., Inc. pp 279-280, 1978.
6. Gikonyo BM, Dunnigan A, Benson DW Jr.: Cardiovascular collapse in infants: Association with paroxysmal atrial tachycardia. *Pediatrics* 76:922, 1985.
7. Garson A Jr: Supraventricular tachycardia, in Gillette PC, Garson A Jr (eds): *Pediatric Cardiac Dysrhythmias.* New York, Grune and Stratton, 1981.
8. Radford D: Side effects of verapamil in infants. *Arch Dis Child* 58:465, 1983.
9. Epstein ML, Kiel EA, Victorica BE: Cardiac decompensation following verapamil therapy in infants with supraventricular tachycardia. *Pediatrics* 75:737, 1985.
10. Walsh CK, Krongrad E: Terminal cardiac electrical activity in pediatric patients. *Am J Cardiol* 51:557, 1983.
11. Eisenberg M, Bergner L, Hallstrom A: Epidemiology of cardiac arrest and resuscitation in children. *Ann Emerg Med* 12:672, 1983.
12. Chameides L, Brown GE, Raye JR, et al: Guidelines for defibrillation in infants and children: Report of the American Heart Association Target Activity Group: Cardiopulmonary resuscitation in the young. *Circulation* 56(suppl):502A, 1977.

Neonatal Resuscitation

The ideal environment for neonatal resuscitation is the delivery room or the neonatal intensive care unit. In these settings, problems can be anticipated, and trained personnel as well as appropriate equipment are always available. Resuscitation in the delivery room is dealt with in a separate course; delivery-room and neonatal-intensive-care personnel should take that course.

Unfortunately, many deliveries occur outside the delivery room — in the home, enroute to the hospital, or in the emergency room, where conditions may be less than optimal. This chapter offers a practical approach to the resuscitation of the neonate, in the peripartum period, in the emergency room or other non-optimal setting, using AHA standards.[1]

I. Triage

Marked changes occur in the cardiovascular and respiratory systems at the moment of birth. The cardiovascular system undergoes a rapid transition from the fetal to the postpartum circulation. The respiratory system, which is essentially nonfunctional *in utero*, must suddenly initiate and maintain the respiratory process. When prepartum events cause asphyxia, they preclude a smooth postpartum transition. The aim of the resuscitative process is restoration of normal cardiopulmonary function.

The vast majority (approximately 80%) of newborn infants require no resuscitation beyond maintenance of temperature, mild stimulation, and suctioning of the airway. Of the small number who require further intervention, most will respond to a high oxygen environment and bag–mask ventilation. A small number of severely asphyxiated infants require chest compression; and an even smaller number, resuscitative medications.

An inverted pyramid (Figure 7.1) illustrates the relative frequencies of performance of the various resuscitative steps. Resuscitation should proceed in a stepwise fashion, with *reassessment* prior to each step, so that complications from unnecessarily aggressive intervention may be avoided.

Since best results are obtained in the most ideal environment, every effort should be made to delay the birth until the mother can be transported to a delivery room. Prehospital delays as well as stops in the emergency room or admitting office are inappropriate.

II. Preparation

Most neonatal resuscitations in the emergency room occur without prior notice. The resuscitative process can, however, be facilitated by preparing equipment and training personnel in advance, by obtaining a brief history, and by assigning personnel prior to, or immediately upon, admission to the emergency room.

A. Advance Preparation

Every emergency department should maintain an easily accessible neonatal resuscitation tray that is periodically checked and replenished. The tray should contain proper equipment (Table 7.1), as well as charts listing the correct medication dosages for neonates of various weights (Table 7.2). Unless equipment is meticulously organized and readily available in the emergency department, even the most sophisticated personnel will find it difficult to perform a successful neonatal resuscitation.

B. Immediate Preparation

As soon as it is evident that a neonatal resuscitation may be necessary, a prearranged plan for assigning personnel according to levels of competence should be put into action. There is usually little time for an in-depth history, but often a brief history reveals key information that may alter the course of the resuscitation. For example, if there is a history of particulate meconium in the amniotic fluid, the resuscitation team must be prepared to suction the trachea under direct vision; if the labor is premature, one can anticipate a probable resuscitation; and if twins are expected, the team must be prepared to resuscitate two infants.

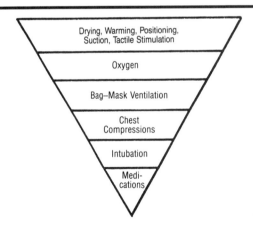

Figure 7.1. Inverted pyramid reflecting the approximate relative frequencies of neonatal resuscitative efforts. Note that a majority of infants respond to simple measures. Most infants requiring chest compression will usually require intubation and these efforts are often performed simultaneously.

Table 7.1. Newborn Resuscitation Equipment for the Emergency Department

A. ITEMS THAT SHOULD BE READILY ACCESSIBLE
   Radiant warmer
   Suction with manometer
   Resuscitation bag (250–500 mL)
   Facemasks (newborn and premature size)
   Laryngoscope with extra battery and bulb
   Laryngoscope blades (straight O and 1)
   Medications
      Epinephrine 1:10,000
      Sodium bicarbonate 4.2%*
      Volume expander
      Naloxone

B. ITEMS THAT SHOULD BE ON NEWBORN RESUSCITATION TRAY
   Bulb syringe
   Mechanical suction device
   Endotracheal tubes (2.5, 3.0, and 3.5)
   Suction catheters (one 5 F and two 8 F each taped
      to the appropriate ET tube)
   Endotracheal tube stylet
   Umbilical catheter (5 Fr)
   Syringe (10 and 20 mL)
   Three-way stopcock
   Feeding tube (5 F and 8 F)
   Towels
   OB kit/cord-cutting materials

*If the adult 8.4% solution is the only one available, it should be diluted 1:1 with sterile water.

When a newborn has been resuscitated prior to arrival at the hospital, special problems include hypothermia and difficulty in maintaining vascular access and airway control during transport. Preparation for receiving the newborn in the emergency department should be similar to preparation for a full resuscitation, and on arrival the newborn should be carefully evaluated.

III. Resuscitation Procedure

A. The Environment

All newborns have difficulty tolerating a cold environment.[2] Asphyxiated infants are particularly at risk, and recovery from acidosis is delayed by hypothermia.[3] Hypothermia may be a special problem for the infant born outside the hospital. Heat loss may be prevented by 1) placing the infant under a preheated warmer and 2) quickly drying the infant of amniotic fluid. A radiant warmer should be switched on as soon as it is known that a neonatal resuscitation may be necessary. Other ways of warming the infant, if a radiant warmer is not available, include using warm towels and placing the naked infant against the body of the mother, with covers over both.

B. Positioning

The newborn should be placed on his/her back in a slight Trendelenburg (head down) position with the neck slightly extended. A 1-inch thickness of blanket or towel placed under the infant's shoulders is helpful in maintaining head position. If copious secretions are present, the infant's head should be turned to the side.

C. Suctioning

To assure an open airway, first the mouth and then the nose should be suctioned. In the emergency room there is frequently insufficient time to adequately adjust the wall suction; in this setting, therefore, manual bulb suction or a mechanical suction device should be available. If a mechanical suction apparatus with an 8 or 10 F suction catheter is used, pressure should not exceed −100 mmHg (−136 cmH$_2$O). Deep suctioning of the oropharynx may produce a vagal response and cause bradycardia and/or apnea.[4] Suctioning should therefore continue for no longer than 10 seconds at a time, and heart rate should be continuously monitored. In order to minimize hypoxia, time should be allowed between suctionings for the lungs to be ventilated, spontaneously or with assistance, with 100% oxygen.

Meconium aspiration is a major cause of neonatal death and morbidity, and its prevention deserves special attention.[5] If meconium is not adequately removed from the airway, a high percent (60%) of infants with thick meconium in the amniotic fluid will aspirate this fluid at the initiation of respiration. Some of these newborns (approximately 20%) will develop complications following meconium aspiration, including respiratory distress, aspiration pneumonia, and pneumothorax.[6] To prevent aspiration, infants born with particulate meconium staining require thorough hypopharyngeal suctioning before initiation of respiration and, therefore, before completion of the delivery.[7] Suctioning should be performed after the head, but not the rest of the body, is delivered. If the hypopharynx has not been cleared of meconium before the onset of respiration, as is likely to happen with a precipitous delivery in the emergency room, the trachea should be intubated to remove as much of the meconium as possible from the lower airway.[8] As meconium is viscous, suction should be applied directly to the endotracheal tube, using the full caliber of the tube to evacuate the thick, tenacious material. Suction catheters inserted through the endotracheal tube are inadequate. The evacuation can be performed by a mechanical suction device. As suction is applied directly to the endotracheal tube, the tube is slowly withdrawn. To facilitate the use of wall suction, the suction control port, removed from a suction catheter, can be attached directly to the endotracheal tube.[9] If meconium is removed via the endotracheal tube, the infant should be reintubated and suctioned again to remove as much meconium as possible. The presence of watery or thin meconium does not require routine endotracheal intubation.

Table 7.2. Neonatal Resusci-Card

Ventilation Rate: 40–60 per minute

Compression Rate: 120 per minute

Medications: Heart rate < 80 per minute despite adequate ventilations with 100% O_2 and chest compressions

Medication	Concentration to Administer	Preparation	Dosage/ Route*	Total Dose/Infant			Rate/Precautions
Epinephrine	1:10,000	1 mL	0.1–0.3 mL/kg IV or ET	weight 1 kg 2 kg 3 kg 4 kg	total mL's 0.1–0.3 mL 0.2–0.6 mL 0.3–0.9 mL 0.4–1.2 mL		Give rapidly
Volume expanders	Whole blood 5% albumin Normal saline Ringer's Lactate	40 mL	10 mL/kg IV	weight 1 kg 2 kg 3 kg 4 kg	total mL's 10 mL 20 mL 30 mL 40 mL		Give over 5–10 min.
Sodium bicarbonate	0.5 mEq/mL (4.2% solution)	20 mL or two 10-mL prefilled syringes	2 mEq/kg IV	weight 1 kg 2 kg 3 kg 4 kg	total dose 2 mEq 4 mEq 6 mEq 8 mEq	total mL's 4 mL 8 mL 12 mL 16 mL	Give slowly over at least 2 minutes Give only if infant being effectively ventilated
Naloxone	0.4 mg/mL or 1.0 mg/mL	1 mL	0.1 mg/kg IV IM SQ ET	weight 1 kg 2 kg 3 kg 4 kg	total dose 0.1 mg 0.2 mg 0.3 mg 0.4 mg		Give rapidly
Dopamine	$6 \times \dfrac{\text{weight (kg)} \times \text{desired dose } (\mu g/kg/min)}{\text{desired fluid (mL/hr)}} = \dfrac{\text{mg of dopamine per 100 mL solution}}{}$		Begin at 5 μg/kg/min (may increase to 20 μg/kg/min if necessary) IV	weight 1 kg 2 kg 3 kg 4 kg	total μg/min 5–20 μg/min. 10–40 μg/min. 15–60 μg/min. 20–80 μg/min.		Give as an infusion using an infusion pump Monitor HR and BP closely Seek consultation

ET/Suction Catheter			
Weight	ET/Catheter	Laryng. Blade	
1 kg	2.5/5F	0	
2 kg	3.0/6F	0	
3 kg	3.5/8F	0–1	
4 kg	3.5/8F	1	

*IM = intramuscular.
ET = endotracheal tube
IV = intravenous
SQ = subcutaneous

D. Tactile Stimulation

Drying and suctioning produce enough stimulation to induce effective respirations in most infants. Two additional safe methods of providing tactile stimulation are 1) slapping or flicking the soles of the feet, and 2) rubbing the infant's back. More vigorous methods of stimulation should be avoided. If the infant fails to establish spontaneous and effective respirations following a brief period of stimulation, positive-pressure ventilation is required.

E. Assessment

If the infant is born in the emergency room, the assessment is performed after clearing the airway and stimulating the infant. If, however, the delivery takes place before arrival in the emergency room, the assessment should be performed immediately after placing the infant in a warmed environment.

1. Respiratory Effort

Breathing rate and depth should increase immediately with *brief* stimulation; time should not be taken to stimulate the infant more than twice.

If the respiratory response is appropriate, the heart rate is evaluated next. If the respiratory response is inappropriate (shallow, slow, or absent respirations), positive-pressure ventilations should be started immediately. Continued tactile stimulation of an apneic infant increases hypoxemia and delays the onset of needed ventilation.

2. Heart Rate

The heart rate is a critical determinant of the resuscitation sequence and may be evaluated by 1) listening to the apical beat with a stethoscope, 2) feeling the pulse by lightly grasping the base of the umbilical cord, or 3) by feeling the brachial or femoral pulse. A cardiotachometer monitoring system can also be used but takes time to set up.

The presence of respirations does not guarantee an adequate pulse rate. Shallow respirations may primarily ventilate airway dead space and thus provide inadequate alveolar ventilation.

If the heart rate is > 100 beats/min and spontaneous respirations are present, the assessment is continued. If the heart rate is < 100 beats/min, positive-pressure ventilations should be started immediately.

3. Color

An infant may occasionally be cyanotic despite adequate ventilations and a heart rate > 100 beats/min. If central cyanosis is present in an infant with spontaneous respirations and an adequate heart rate, free-flow oxygen should be given until the cause can be further evaluated. Oxygen therapy is unnecessary for infants with peripheral cyanosis (blue extremities only), a condition common in the first few minutes of life and due to sluggish peripheral circulation.

4. The Apgar Score

The Apgar scoring system (Table 7.3) has been widely used as an indicator of the need for resuscitation at birth. Five objective signs are evaluated, and the total score is noted at 1 minute and at 5 minutes after the complete birth of the infant. If the 5-minute Apgar score is less than 7, additional scores are obtained every 5 minutes for a total of 20 minutes. The need for resuscitation can, however, be more rapidly assessed by evaluating the *heart rate, respiratory activity,* and *color* than by the total Apgar score. Since even a short delay in initiating resuscitation may result in a long delay in establishing spontaneous and regular respirations, resuscitation should be started immediately when indicated by inadequate respirations and/or heart rate. It should not be delayed while obtaining the one-minute score.

Table 7.3. Apgar Scoring

Sign	0	1	2
Heart rate	Absent	Slow (< 100/min)	> 100/min
Respirations	Absent	Slow, irregular	Good, crying
Muscle tone	Limp	Some flexion	Active motion
Reflex irritability (catheter in nares)	No response	Grimace	Cough or sneeze
Color	Blue or pale	Pink body with blue extremities	Completely pink

F. Ventilation

The vast majority of infants who require ventilatory support may be adequately ventilated using a bag and mask. Indications for positive-pressure ventilation include 1) apnea, 2) heart rate < 100 beats/min, and 3) persistent central cyanosis in a maximal oxygen environment.

An assisted ventilatory rate of 40–60 breaths/min should provide adequate ventilation. Tidal volumes in newborn and, especially, preterm infants are small. To minimize the chance of possible iatrogenic complications, it is best to begin bag–mask ventilations with small volumes, increasing rapidly, though in small increments, until an adequate tidal volume is achieved. It is imperative to maintain a tight face mask seal for adequate ventilations. In most infants, initial lung inflation requires pressures of 30–40 cmH_2O; in some, pressures as high as 60 cmH_2O may be needed; less pressure is usually required for succeeding breaths. Signs of adequate ventilation include bilateral expansion of the lungs as judged by chest wall motion and auscultation of breath sounds. Inability to inflate the lungs adequately requires further suctioning and repositioning of the head and face mask. If these maneuvers fail to provide adequate ventilation, immediate laryngoscopic examination of the upper airway and intubation of the trachea is required. Bag and mask ventilation may produce gastric distention requiring periodic decompression. If bag–mask positive-pressure ventilations are required for longer than approximately 2 minutes, an orogastric tube should be inserted into the stomach and left in place during ventilations.

After adequate ventilation has been established for 15–30 seconds, subsequent steps depend on the heart rate. If the heart rate is > 100 beats/min and spontaneous respirations are present, positive-pressure ventilation may be discontinued. Gentle tactile stimulation, such as rubbing the baby's skin, may help to maintain spontane–

ous breathing. If there are no spontaneous respirations, assisted ventilation must be continued.

If, despite adequate ventilations, the heart rate is < 60 beats/min or 60–80 beats/min and not rapidly increasing, positive–pressure–assisted ventilations should be continued and chest compressions initiated.

1. Ventilation Bags

Self-Inflating Bag: Many of the self-inflating bags are equipped with a pressure-limited pop-off valve that is usually preset at 30–35 cmH$_2$O. Since the first breaths of a neonate's nonaerated lung may require higher pressures, this feature may prevent initial effective inflation unless the pop-off valve is occluded. Self-inflating bags that have a device to bypass the pop-off valve and an in-line manometer are preferred. Bag volumes should not exceed 750 mL; larger bags make it difficult to accurately provide the small tidal volumes that infants require. (See also Chapter 3.)

Anesthesia Bag: The anesthesia bag inflates only when air or oxygen from a compressed gas source is forced into it. It requires a well-modulated flow of gas into the inlet port, correct adjustment of the flow control valve, and careful attention to a tight seal at the face mask. Since an anesthesia bag can deliver very high pressures, a port with an attached pressure gauge must be present to monitor peak ventilatory pressures. The anesthesia bag requires more training in its proper use than a self-inflating bag. (See also Chapter 3.)

2. Face Masks

Face masks have either cushioned or noncushioned rims and are round or anatomically shaped. Anatomically shaped masks are designed to fit the contours of the infant's face and have a low dead space (< 5 mL). The anatomical shape and cushioned rim provide the greatest chance for making a tight seal, and they help avoid mispositioning the mask. A correctly positioned mask should cover the infant's nose and mouth but not the eyes. Face masks fitting preterm, term, and large newborns should be available on the neonatal resuscitation tray.

3. Endotracheal Intubation

Endotracheal intubation is indicated if:

1. bag–mask ventilation is ineffective;
2. tracheal suctioning is required, especially for thick meconium; or
3. prolonged positive-pressure ventilation is necessary.

The supplies and equipment for endotracheal intubation should be kept together and readily available on the neonatal resuscitation tray. Sterile, disposable tubes of nonirritating material should be used. Those designated IT (implantation tested) or Z79 meet the required standards. Tubes with a uniform internal diameter are

preferred to those that are tapered. Most endotracheal tubes intended for neonatal use have a black line guide — vocal cord line — near the tip. If this guide is placed at the cord level, the tip of the tube is likely to be above the carina. The endotracheal tube size required is related to the infant's weight. (Table 7.2).

The position of the endotracheal tube may be checked by 1) observing for symmetrical chest wall motion and listening for equal breath sounds, especially at the apices, and 2) if the tube is to remain in place following the resuscitation, a chest roentgenogram.

G. Chest Compressions

Asphyxia causes tissue hypoxia, acidosis, poor myocardial contractility, bradycardia, and eventually, cardiac arrest. This critical state can often be avoided by prompt and effective ventilation and oxygenation. Chest compressions should be performed if the heart rate is < 60 beats/min or 60–80 beats/min and not rapidly increasing despite adequate ventilation with 100% oxygen for approximately 30 seconds.

There are two techniques for performing chest compressions in the neonate and small infant. One[10] employs both thumbs placed on the lower third of the sternum, with the fingers encircling the torso and supporting the back (Figure 7.2). The thumbs should be positioned side-by-side on the sternum just below a line between the two nipples. In the very small infant the thumbs may have to

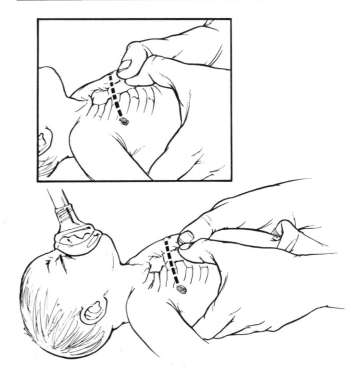

Figure 7.2. Hand position for chest encirclement technique for external chest compressions in neonates. Thumbs are side-by-side over the midsternum. In the small newborn, thumbs may need to be superimposed.

be superimposed. Because of the potential for damaging the abdominal organs, the xiphoid portion of the sternum should not be compressed.

If the infant is large or the resuscitator's hands are too small to encircle the chest, two-finger compressions with the ring and middle fingers on the sternum one finger's breadth below the nipple line, but not over the xiphoid, are applied (see Chapter 2). The sternum is compressed ½ to ¾ inches at a rate of 120 times/min. The compression phase should be smooth, not jerky, and equal in time to the relaxation phase. The thumbs or fingers should not be lifted off the sternum during the relaxation phase. The pulse rate should be checked periodically and chest compressions discontinued when the spontaneous heart rate reaches 80 beats/min or greater. Compressions should always be accompanied by positive-pressure ventilations with 100% oxygen at a rate of 40–60 breaths/min.

H. Medications and Fluids

Myocardial dysfunction and shock in the neonatal period are usually the result of profound hypoxia. Medications should be administered if, despite adequate ventilation with 100% oxygen and chest compressions for 30 seconds, there is no heart rate or the heart rate remains < 80 beats/min.

There is no current evidence that two previously recommended drugs, atropine and calcium, are useful in the acute phase of neonatal resuscitation. Sodium bicarbonate may be useful in a prolonged resuscitation to help correct metabolic acidosis[11] but should not be used in brief arrests or episodes of bradycardia.[12–16] In the absence of adequate ventilation, sodium bicarbonate will not improve blood pH. Hypoxemia and acidosis may best be corrected with adequate oxygenation and ventilation.

1. Routes of Administration

The umbilical vein is preferred for vascular access during neonatal resuscitation because the vessel is easily located and cannulated, but the catheter is usually withdrawn at the end of the resuscitation to minimize the danger of infection or portal vein thrombosis.

The cord is trimmed with a scalpel blade 1 cm above the skin attachment and held firmly to prevent bleeding. The umbilical vein is recognized as a thin-walled single vessel, in contrast to the arteries, which are paired, thicker walled, and often constricted. The vein lumen is larger than that of the artery, so the vessel that continues to bleed after the cord is cut is usually the vein. A 5.0 F umbilical catheter with a radiopaque marker, attached to a three-way stopcock and filled with saline, is inserted so that the tip is just below the skin and there is free flow of blood; the catheter is inserted a short distance to avoid inadvertent infusion of hypertonic solutions into the liver. A wedged hepatic position is recognized by failure of free blood return. If this occurs, the catheter should be withdrawn to a position where blood can be freely aspirated.

Vascular access via other routes may also be obtained. Cannulating the umbilical artery is more time consuming and difficult, but it is useful for monitoring blood pressure, blood gases, and acid–base balance. Fluids and most medications may be given via this route. Peripheral veins in the extremities and scalp are difficult to access in neonates during a resuscitation.

When venous access is not readily available, the endotracheal tube is the most easily accessible route for delivery of epinephrine[17,18] and should eliminate the need for intracardiac injections. Since the optimal dose for the endotracheal route is currently not certain,[19] the intravenous dose is recommended.[20,21] It is advisable to dilute the medication in 1–2 mL of normal saline and to deliver it via a feeding tube passed into the endotracheal tube so that the medication is delivered into the trachea.

2. Epinephrine (see Chapter 5)

Indications: Asystole or spontaneous heart rate < 80 beats/min despite adequate ventilation with 100% oxygen and chest compressions.

Dose: 0.01–0.03 mg/kg (0.1–0.3 mL/kg of the 1:10,000 solution). May be repeated every 5 minutes if required.

Route: Intravenously or via endotracheal tube.

3. Volume Expanders

Volume expanders are indicated in the presence of hypovolemia, which should be suspected in any infant who requires resuscitation.

Indications: Evidence of acute bleeding from the fetal–maternal unit with 1) pallor that persists after oxygenation, 2) faint pulses with a good heart rate, and 3) poor response to resuscitation with adequate ventilation.

Dose: 1) 10 mL/kg O-negative blood cross matched with the mother's blood; 2) 10 mL/kg 5% albumin/saline solution or other plasma substitute; or 3) 10 mL/kg normal saline or Ringer's lactate. Volume expanders are given over 5–10 minutes.

Route: Intravenously.

4. Sodium Bicarbonate (see Chapter 5)

Indications: Acidosis accompanying cardiac arrest is best treated with hyperventilation. Sodium bicarbonate may be used in a prolonged arrest unresponsive to other medications or if profound metabolic acidosis is documented, but it should not be used in brief episodes of bradycardia or arrest.

Dose: 2 mEq/kg of a 4.2% solution (4 mL/kg; 0.5 mEq/mL). If only the 1.0 mEq/mL solution is available, it should be diluted with an equal amount of sterile water.

Route: Intravenously (by slow push).

5. Dopamine (see Chapter 5)

Occasionally, a dopamine infusion may be needed. This drug is discussed in Chapter 5, and the dosing regimen is given in Table 7.2.

6. Naloxone Hydrochloride

Naloxone hydrochloride is a narcotic antagonist without direct respiratory effects.

Indications: For the reversal of respiratory depression in the neonate induced by a variety of narcotics given to the mother within 4 hours of delivery. Prompt and adequate ventilatory assistance should always precede the administration of naloxone. Since the duration of action of narcotics may exceed that of naloxone, continued surveillance of the infant is necessary. Naloxone can induce a withdrawal reaction in an infant of a narcotic-addicted mother and should be used with caution if this condition is suspected.

Dose: 0.1 mg/kg (0.1 mL/kg of 1.0 mg/mL dosage or 0.25 mL/kg of 0.4 mg/mL dosage). The initial dose may be repeated every 2 to 3 minutes as needed.

Route: Intravenously, via the endotracheal tube or, if perfusion is adequate, subcutaneously or intramuscularly.

IV. Postresuscitation Care

Some emergency departments, especially those located in rural areas, may receive infants born outside the hospital who have already been resuscitated. An infant who has been resuscitated prior to arrival at the hospital should be assumed to have an airway problem. Some of the more common complications include dislodgement or endobronchial displacement of the endotracheal tube during transport, endotracheal tube occlusion by mucous or meconium, and pneumothorax. The latter can be especially difficult to diagnose by auscultation, since breath sounds in the neonate may be transmitted. A diagnosis of pneumothorax should be considered in a newborn who deteriorates after an initial response or who fails to respond to resuscitative efforts.

Communication with a neonatal intensive care unit should be established as soon as it is known that there is a potential neonatal resuscitation. Postresuscitation care, while still in the emergency room, may include determination of arterial blood gases, correction of documented metabolic acidosis, treatment of hypotension with volume expanders and/or inotropic agents, and treatment of seizures, hypoglycemia, and hypocalcemia. A chest roentgenogram helps to rule out a pneumothorax and demonstrate the location of the endotracheal tube.

After successful resuscitation the infant should be monitored closely by trained observers in an intensive care area.

References

1. Standards and Guidelines for Cardiopulmonary Resuscitation (CPR) and Emergency Cardiac Care (ECC) *JAMA* 255:2969, 1986.
2. Scopes JW, Ahmed I: Range of critical temperatures in sick and premature newborn babies. *Arch Dis Child* 41:417, 1966.
3. Adamsons K Jr, Gandy GM, James LS: The influence of thermal factors upon oxygen consumption of the newborn human infant. *J Pediatr* 66:495, 1965.
4. Cordero L, Hon EH: Neonatal bradycardia following nasopharyngeal stimulation. *J Pediatr* 78:441, 1971.
5. Carson BS, Losey RW, Bowes WA Jr, et al: Combined obstetric and pediatric approach to prevent meconium aspiration syndrome. *Am J Obstet Gynecol* 126:712, 19765.
6. Fox WW, Gutsche BB, DeVore JS: A delivery room approach to the meconium aspiration syndrome (MAS). Immediate intubation, endotracheal suction, and oxygen administration can reduce morbidity and mortality. *Clin Pediatr* 16:325, 1977.
7. Gregory GA, Gooding CA, Phibbs RH, et al: Meconium aspiration in infants — A prospective study. *J Pediatr* 85:848, 1974.
8. Ting P, Brady JP: Tracheal suction in meconium aspiration. *Am J Obstet Gynecol* 122:767, 1975.
9. Eisner P: Suctioning meconium from the trachea: A new solution to an old problem. *Pediatrics* 78:713, 1986.
10. Todres ID, Rogers MC: Methods of external cardiac massage in the newborn infant. *J Pediatr* 86:781, 1975.
11. Bishop RL, Weisfeldt MC: Sodium bicarbonate administration during cardiac arrest: Effect on arterial pH, PCO_2 and osmolality. *JAMA* 235: 506, 1976.
12. Ostrea EM, Odell GB: The influence of bicarbonate administration on blood pH in a "closed system:" Clinical implications. *J Pediatr* 80:671, 1972.
13. Simmons MA, Adock EW III, Bard H, et al: Hypernatremia and intracranial hemorrhage in neonates. *N Engl J Med* 291:6, 1974.
14. Finberg L: The relationship of intravenous infusions and intracranial hemorrhage — A commentary. *J Pediatr* 91:777, 1977.
15. Papile LA, Bursetin J, Burstein R, et al: Relationship of intravenous sodium bicarbonate infusions and cerebral intraventricular hemorrhage. *J Pediatr* 93:834, 1978.
16. Graf H, Leach W, Arieff AI: Evidence for a detrimental effect of bicarbonate therapy in lactic acidosis. *Science* 227:754, 1985.
17. Greenberg MI, Roberts JR, Baskin SI, et al: The use of endotracheal medication for cardiac arrest. *Top Emerg Med* 1:29, 1979.
18. Ward JT Jr: Endotracheal drug therapy. *Am J Emerg Med* 1:71, 1983.
19. Lindemann R: Endotracheal administration of epinephrine during cardiopulmonary resuscitation (letter). *Am J Dis Child* 136:753, 1982.
20. Roberts JR, Greenberg MI, Knaub MA, et al: Comparison of the pharmacological effects of epinephrine administered by the intravenous and endotracheal routes. *JACEP* 7:260, 1978.
21. Roberts JR, Greenberg MI, Knaub MA, et al: Blood levels following intravenous and endotracheal epinephrine administration. *JACEP* 8:53, 1979.

Immediate Postarrest Stabilization

Chapter 8

Postresuscitation care involves patient stabilization, transport to a tertiary care facility, and ongoing care within such a facility. The latter encompasses the entire discipline of pediatric intensive care; this chapter deals with immediate postarrest stabilization and the care needed during transport.

The goal of postarrest stabilization and transport is to avoid secondary organ injury and to have the patient arrive at a tertiary care setting in the best possible physiologic state. The airway should be secured and ventilation carefully assessed. Frequent examination of peripheral perfusion and organ function is essential to uncover early signs of organ dysfunction and thus permit early therapy. A system that establishes good communication between the referring and accepting hospitals can improve patient outcome.

I. General Care

Any infant or child requiring resuscitation from a respiratory or cardiac arrest, no matter how good the initial response to resuscitation, should have repeated and regular cardiopulmonary assessments (see Chapter 1) and should be transferred to a pediatric intensive care unit for further observation and care.

General postresuscitation care prior to and during transport includes the following:

1. Regular and repeated cardiopulmonary assessments (see Chapter 1), including the following:
   a. Continuous ECG monitoring of heart rate and rhythm.
   b. Blood pressure recording, directly by intraarterial cannula, or indirectly by a Doppler measuring device or sphygmomanometer every 5 minutes until stable, and every 15 minutes thereafter.
   c. Evaluation of peripheral circulation and end-organ perfusion, including skin temperature, capillary refill, quality of distal pulses, level of consciousness, and urine output. The latter can best be monitored with an indwelling Foley catheter.
   d. Evaluation of ventilation by observing chest motion, use of accessory muscles, nasal flaring, auscultation of lung fields, and interpretation of arterial blood gases. Continuous noninvasive monitoring of oxygenation (by pulse oximeter or transcutaneous pO_2) is helpful in preventing episodes of hypoxemia.
   e. Serial neurologic examinations with special attention to the onset of intracranial hypertension or seizures. These may affect ventilation if chest wall rigidity or apnea develop.

2. Humidified oxygen at the highest attainable concentration until objective assessment by an arterial blood gas analysis indicates that less oxygen is needed.
3. Two well-secured and functioning intravenous lines. The following are guidelines for initial maintenance fluids (special circumstances may dictate a different type or rate of solution):
   - For an infant < 10 kg: an infusion of $D_{10}W$ with ¼% NS, at a rate of 4 mL/kg/hr.
   - For a child 10–20 kg: an infusion of D_5W with ¼% NS, at a rate of 40 mL/hr + 2 mL/kg/hr for kg > 10; e.g., maintenance rate for a 15-kg child is 40 + (2 × 5) = 50 mL/hr.
   - For a child > 20 kg: an infusion of D_5W in ¼% NS, at a rate of 40 + 1 mL/kg/hr; e.g., maintenance fluids for a 30-kg child is 40 + 30 = 70 mL/hr.
4. Blood studies determined by specific circumstances, but usually arterial blood gases, electrolytes, calcium, glucose, and hematocrit. Arterial blood gas analysis, after at least a 15-minute period of equilibration on the ventilating system to be used during transport, should be repeated, if feasible, just prior to transport.
5. A nasogastric tube to gravity drainage, which is useful to keep the stomach decompressed, especially in patients receiving positive-pressure ventilation, and is almost always indicated in critically ill children, especially if they are obtunded.
6. A search for the precipitating cause of the arrest and appropriate therapy (e.g., antibiotics) should be started.
7. Careful attention to preserving core temperature. This is especially, but not exclusively, important in infants. Prior to transport, overhead heating units can be used for infants; and heating lamps, for children. During transport, portable incubators are useful for infants; older children should be covered, especially the head, which represents a relatively large portion of the body surface.

II. Special Care for Patients With Organ Failure

In the immediate postresuscitation period, many children have hypoxemia and/or hypercapnea, hemodynamic instability, and/or an an altered sensorium.

A. Respiratory System

Failure of any component of the respiratory system is both a common cause and a result of cardiopulmonary arrest. When hemodynamic stability permits cessation of chest compressions, manual ventilations may be replaced by mechanical ventilation, but if mechanical ventilation is not available, manual ventilation with bag and endotracheal tube can be continued throughout the transport.

Elective intubation should be considered for any infant or child at risk of respiratory or cardiovascular embarrassment. The endotracheal tube must be securely taped and its position confirmed by chest x-ray. This cannot be stressed enough since it may be very difficult, en route, to recognize dislodgement of the endotracheal tube and even more difficult to reintubate the child. Agitated children may need to be sedated, and muscle relaxants are sometimes required to minimize accidental tube dislodgement during transport. Commonly used sedatives are diazepam (0.1–0.2 mg/kg IV) and morphine sulphate (0.1 mg/kg IV). Muscle paralysis may be achieved with pancuronium bromide (0.1 mg/kg IV). Mechanical or manual ventilation must be provided since narcotics, sedatives, and muscle relaxants reduce or ablate the ventilatory drive.

The following guidelines are suggested beginning settings for mechanical ventilation. Adequacy of ventilation and oxygenation should be verified by arterial blood gases.

1. Initial Ventilator Settings

(See Table 8.1.)

Oxygen: Low cardiac output promotes intrapulmonary right-to-left shunting. Since the risks of hyperoxia over a brief period are negligible compared with the risks of inadequate tissue oxygenation, the *initial* FiO_2 should be 1.0 even in the presence of a high arterial oxygen tension.

Tidal Volume: When a volume ventilator is used, delivered tidal volume should initially be set at 10–15 mL/kg. If there is a large air leak around the endotracheal tube, susbstantially higher volumes are required; the endotracheal tube may need to be replaced with a larger one. Adequacy of tidal volume is assessed by a good chest expansion, good breath sounds, and a normal $PaCO_2$. For most patients inspiratory time should be at least 0.5 seconds.

Peak Inspiratory Pressure: When a timed-cycled, pressure-limited ventilator is used, the peak inspiratory pressure setting should be adjusted according to the size of the patient and the disease process. Infants and children with normal lung compliance are usually well ventilated at peak inspiratory pressures of 20–30 cmH_2O and inspiratory times of 0.5–1.0 seconds. Higher pressures are required in the presence of lung disease. Initial peak inspiratory pressure should be set at the lowest level that provides adequate chest expansion and good breath sounds.

Similar peak inspiratory pressures are usually generated with volume ventilators, when 10–15 mL/kg tidal volumes are delivered. When using volume-limited ventilation, the pressure limit alarm should be set about 10 cmH_2O higher than the peak inspiratory pressure in order to protect against barotrauma and provide warning of a sudden increase in airway resistance (i.e., accidentally occluded endotracheal tube, pneumothorax, or mainstem bronchus intubation). Volume ventilation is preferred since a preset tidal volume will be delivered even if the endotracheal tube is partly occluded.

Respiratory Rate: In the absence of lung disease, infants commonly require a respiratory rate of 20–30 breaths/min. Older children require a slower rate, about 16–20 breaths/min. In the presence of lung disease, higher rates are usually required to achieve adequate ventilation, although in certain situations a slower ventilation rate is indicated, even when elevated CO_2 is documented. Specifically, when the patient has asthma, bronchiolitis, or other conditions causing air trapping, rapid ventilation rates may not provide adequate time for exhalation; breaths will then stack and the patient will be at high risk for developing a pneumothorax. Auscultation will determine when exhalation is ending relative to the next breath. In general, such patients require a tidal volume of 15 mL/kg delivered slowly (rates of 20–25 breaths/min in infants and 8–12 breaths/minute in adolescents) with adequate time for exhalation. It is particularly helpful in these patients with small airway trapping to use muscle relaxants since the patients' respiratory efforts often worsen airway obstruction.

Positive End-Expiratory Pressure (PEEP): Intubation bypasses glottic function. In order to maintain adequate functional residual capacity, 3–5 cmH_2O PEEP should be provided when mechanical ventilation is initiated. Higher levels may be therapeutic if oxygenation is inadequate because of diffuse alveolar disease or marked ventilation/perfusion mismatch.

Table 8.1. Initial Ventilator Settings

These initial ventilator settings should be adjusted according to clinical state and arterial blood gas monitoring.

Oxygen	100%
Tidal volume	10–15 mL/kg
Inspiratory time	≥ 0.5 seconds
Peak inspiratory pressure	20–30 cmH_2O with normal lung compliance (lowest level that gives adequate chest expansion)
Respiratory rate	Infants: 20–30 breaths/min. Children: 16–20 breaths/min.
PEEP	3–5 cmH_2O

2. Assessment of Ventilation and Oxygenation Following Intubation

Inspection provides valuable clues about respiratory effort in mechanically ventilated children. Tachypnea, head bobbing, nasal flaring, retractions, and the use of accessory neck and abdominal muscles indicate increased work of breathing. Agitation may reflect inadequate oxygenation or ventilation, while cyanosis of the mucous membranes is a clear indication of hypoxemia, although hypoxemia may occur in the absence of overt cyanosis (see Chapter 1).

Chest wall movement and breath sounds should be equal bilaterally. Careful auscultation over the lateral lung fields is important in avoiding confusion from transmitted central airway sounds. Unilateral breath sounds, especially on the right, raise the possibility of right mainstem bronchus intubation but may also be caused by a mucous plug, foreign body obstruction, pneumothorax, pleural effusion, or lung consolidation. Rales, rhonchi, or wheezing may be heard in the presence of pulmonary edema, infection, aspiration, or bronchospasm.

Endotracheal tube position can be determined with certainty from a chest x-ray. The tip should lie 1–2 cm above the carina and below the clavicles.

Adequacy of ventilation and oxygenation is determined by careful patient observation and correct interpretation of arterial blood gas analysis. Resolution of cyanosis and return of pink color reflect improvement in oxygenation. A visible chest rise with positive-pressure ventilation and good breath sounds is suggestive of an adequate tidal volume. Continued patient efforts to breathe against the ventilator may point to an inadequate minute ventilation.

Arterial blood for gas analysis should be obtained 10–15 minutes after initiation of mechanical ventilation. Samples may be obtained from the radial, temporal, posterior tibial, dorsalis pedis, or femoral arteries (see Chapter 4). If arterial puncture is unsuccessful, a capillary sample may be obtained from the heel, toe, or finger after the extremity has been warmed for 15 minutes. If blood flows freely, a reasonably accurate reflection of acid–base status and $PaCO_2$ is obtained, although the PaO_2 may be underestimated. If blood flow is sluggish, all aspects of the gas analysis are potentially unreliable. Noninvasive monitoring devices, including pulse oximeters and transcutaneous O_2 and CO_2 monitors, provide continuous assessment of oxygenation and ventilation but may be inaccurate in the presence of hypothermia or poor peripheral perfusion, problems commonly seen in postresuscitation patients.

B. Cardiovascular System

Circulatory failure may be either the cause or the result of the cardiopulmonary arrest. Persistent circulatory dysfunction is likely in the postresuscitation phase, and cardiac output must be supported to assure adequate oxygen delivery to tissues.

When hemodynamic stability permits cessation of chest compressions, a rapid assessment of cardiovascular function should be performed (see Chapter 1). Prevention of recurrent cardiopulmonary arrest depends on improving the hemodynamic status, based on frequent cardiovascular assessments and appropriate therapeutic interventions, before irreversible changes occur. Evidence of decreased cardiac output or shock may be due to insufficient volume resuscitation, loss of peripheral vascular tone (as seen in septic, anaphylactic, or neurogenic shock), or myocardial dysfunction with inadequate, or premature, withdrawal of support (see Chapter 5).

Children who have experienced a cardiac or respiratory arrest should have continuous monitoring of heart rate and rhythm until extended stability is demonstrated (see Chapter 6). Blood pressure must be measured frequently, keeping in mind that normotension does not assure an adequate cardiac output and that hypotension demands urgent therapy (see Chapter 1). In children with intense vasoconstriction, Korotkoff sounds may be difficult to hear, and systolic pressure may be better measured by palpation or with a Doppler device. As soon as practical, direct arterial monitoring should be instituted in patients with compromised cardiovascular function.

If central venous access has been established and facilities are available, continuous or intermittent right heart filling pressure measurement may help guide therapeutic intervention.

Laboratory evaluation of the circulatory state includes arterial blood gas analysis, serum electrolytes, calcium, glucose, urea nitrogen, and creatinine levels. The presence of metabolic acidosis suggests that the circulatory state is inadequate. Chest x-ray evaluation of heart size may help determine intravascular volume; a small heart is consistent with hypovolemia and a large heart, in the absence of abnormal cardiac function, with volume overload.

C. Central Nervous System

Central nervous system dysfunction may be the cause or result of a cardiopulmonary arrest. If there is evidence of serious central nervous system depression (see Chapter 1), it is safest to intubate the patient and maintain the $PaCO_2$ at 25–30 mmHg until intracranial pressure status can be more completely evaluated. Maintenance of blood pressure and perfusion is essential to assure adequate cerebral perfusion pressure.

III. Pediatric Transport System

Every pediatric tertiary care facility should be part of an organized pediatric transport system. Such a system is usually regionalized, with central control at a pediatric tertiary care facility, under the direction of a physician trained in pediatric emergency or critical care. Transportation of a critically ill infant or child is best performed by a team experienced in the transport and care of such children, even if this causes a delay at the referring institution. The transport team should be capable of delivering advanced pediatric life support at the referring hospital and of maintaining that level of care during transport.

Part of the responsibility of both the referring facility and the tertiary care unit is to establish well-defined protocols dealing with specific clinical situations. Protocols for transporting pediatric patients directly to hospitals and facilities equipped to handle their critical care needs should be included in Emergency Medical System protocols in order to avoid a second transport.[1,2]

A. Interhospital Communication

Early communication between the referring and tertiary care facilities is critical to the success of a transport system. The following information should be transmitted;

- The child's name, age, and weight.
- A description of the child's current illness and significant past medical history, including home and hospital medications.
- The child's present clinical state, including *measured* heart rate, respiratory rate, blood pressure, and temperature, as well as assessment of capillary refill and distal pulses.
- Key laboratory data, especially a recent arterial blood gas.
- The number of intravenous lines, fluid type, and infusion rate.
- Ventilator settings.

A transport medical record should be completed (see Appendix B) and should include a legible copy of the history, physical findings, laboratory data, medications, response to therapy, current clinical findings, name and telephone number of the referring and family physicians, and the name(s) and telephone number(s) of a family member(s). Vital sign flow sheets, nurse's notes, and a copy of all x-rays should accompany the patient.

B. Method of Transport[3]

Transport may take place via surface ambulance, helicopter, or fixed-wing aircraft. Each system has advantages and disadvantages, many of which depend on local conditions. Helicopter cabins tend to be crowded, cannot be pressurized, and have vibrations and noise that make auscultatory monitoring difficult. Fixed-wing aircraft can be partially (620 mmHg) or fully pressurized. Atmospheric pressure decreases as altitude increases (at sea level atmospheric pressure = 760 mmHg; at 5,000 ft = 620 mmHg; at 35,000 ft = 176 mmHg). This results in decreased alveolar pO_2 in ambient air and the expansion of gases in body cavities, such as the stomach or pleural space (pneumothorax), at higher altitudes. Air pressure in the cuff of an endotracheal tube needs to be adjusted

(decreased at higher altitudes and increased when landing). Battery-operated intravenous infusion pumps are more reliable than gravity drip methods for accurately administering fluids at high altitudes.

References

1. Boyd D: Comprehensive regional trauma and emergency medical delivery systems: A goal of the 1980's. *Crit Care Q* 5:11, 1982.
2. Haller JA Jr, Shorter N, Miller D, et al.: Organization and function of a regional pediatric trauma center: Does a system of management improve outcome? *J Trauma* 23:691, 1983.
3. Guidelines for air and ground transportation of pediatric patients. American Academy of Pediatrics Committee on Hospital Care. *Pediatrics* 78: 943, 1986.

Chapter 9

Ethical and Legal Aspects of Cardiopulmonary Resuscitation in Children

In the two decades since the introduction of external chest compression,[1] cardiopulmonary resuscitation (CPR) has gained acceptance as an effective emergency technique that can significantly reduce mortality and be mastered readily by both professionals and laypersons. Organized efforts to encourage this mastery by larger numbers via hospital- and community-based programs have established CPR as a standard treatment modality with attendant legal and ethical issues.

The search for principles to guide the conduct of potential rescuers in these dramatic encounters with sudden death is part of the larger, continuing exploration of the impact of modern medical technology on the traditional patient–provider relationship. Of particular relevance is the continuing evolution of the position of children in our society, their legal standing, and the legal predicates of the special relationships among provider, parent, and child in the pediatric healthcare setting.

Ethical analysis of these relationships tests the specific conduct of the individual against the more generalized beliefs, values, and moral principles from which rules applicable to the issues at hand may be derived

Legal analysis entails examination of the relevant *statutory* law or *common* law. Statutory law codifies rules of conduct by legislative act, leaving to the courts the limited task of interpreting legislative intent and statutory meaning in individual cases. In the absence of such statutes, cases may be decided by common law, in which appellate judges rely on past findings of the courts in similar cases. Such court decisions, though often widely publicized, may have only limited precedential value outside their own jurisdictions.

The purpose of this chapter is to present some of the general principles underlying the ethical and legal rights and duties of patients, healthcare providers, and hospitals and to relate those principles specifically to cardiopulmonary resuscitation, highlighting aspects unique to the care of children.

I. The Child as a Patient

Analysis of the features that distinguish pediatric from adult patients begins with a view of the child in a dynamic state of physiologic and psychosocial development, starting with fetal life and continuing through adolescence. These distinctions carry significant ethical and legal, as well as clinical, implications.

The hallmark of pediatric care is the interpretation of clinical data by reference to age-related norms. In contrast to adults, expected normal values for physical and biochemical measurements in children vary predictably with chronologic and developmental age. Appreciation of this phenomenon in the context of assessing vital signs, body gas and fluid exchanges, and responses to medications and dosage levels is essential to the proper application of pediatric CPR.

Similarly, patterns of psychosocial maturation, from the complete dependence of the infant to the full rational/cognitive capacity of the adolescent, imply progressive evolution of the balance of individual rights and obligations among child, guardian, and healthcare providers.

These unique developmental aspects of pediatrics are fundamental to the universal recognition of pediatrics as a specialty area within medicine. Practitioners and hospitals providing care for children are legally judged by widely accepted pediatric standards. It should be anticipated that these specific standards will encompass the quality of resuscitative care and the associated decision-making process in individual cases.

II. The Patient–Physician Relationship

A. Ethical Principles

Throughout much of medical history, physicians have been guided by principles derived from the Hippocratic Oath. The dominant Hippocratic theme calls on physicians to use their knowledge and skills for the benefit of their patients and to protect them from harm. Contemporary writers have noted the absence here of any explicit patient role in the decision-making process. They question whether this paternalistic stance is appropriate in an era when highly invasive technology may blur the line between "benefit" and "harm".[2]

The rights of patients as decision-makers has only recently been recognized in medical professional codes of ethics.[3] The modern view frames the patient–physician relationship as a collaborative process to which the physician contributes medical knowledge, skill, and judgment and the patient provides a personal valuation of the potential benefits and risks inherent in the proposed treatment. This contractual relationship effectuates the important moral principles of individual patient autonomy and his or her right to self-determination.

Issues of patient autonomy, shared decision-making, the dilemmas of balancing benefits and harms are particularly germaine to cardiopulmonary resuscitation and the appropriate application of life support technology in individual cases. They are further complicated in cases involving minors, where highly valued traditions of family privacy and parental authority may be challenged.

B. Legal Issues

Of special relevance to persons finding themselves unexpectedly at the scene of a cardiopulmonary arrest is an appreciation of the legal definitions marking the beginning and end of the patient–physician relationship. There are basically two avenues by which physicians may enter into a legal relationship with a patient. Most commonly, a legal relationship is created by an advance agreement requiring the physician to provide a specific course of treatment in exchange for compensation. More applicable to the CPR context, however, are the legal obligations arising from rendering care without prior agreement. In general, once a physician or other person performs an act that may be construed as rendering care, there follows a legal duty to meet some "reasonable standard" (discussed more fully below) in the performance of that act and to continue the effort.[4] *Once treatment has been undertaken, the legal relationship with a patient may not be unilaterally terminated by the provider unless care is no longer needed, the patient agrees to terminate the relationship, or appropriate procedures for the transfer of care have been carried out.*[5]

C. Consent

Central to the patient–physician relationship is the notion of "consent," a traditional moral and legal concept that has in modern times evolved into a complex codification of patients' rights of self-determination. At first glance, considerations of consent may appear remote from the circumstances of emergency care, where consent to treatment may usually be implied.[6] However, patient interest in directives through which they may prescribe preferred treatment in the event of cardiac arrest, growing numbers of cases in which competent patients refuse consent for further life support treatment, and the frequency with which third parties are called on to serve as proxy decision-makers for incompetent patients suggest the need for familiarity with the basic aspects of this subject.

In his classic assertion that every person of sound mind and mature years has the right to determine what shall happen to his own body,[7] Judge Cardozo defined patients' rights to grant *permission* for treatment, without which a physician may be guilty of committing an assault. Modern legal decisions have elaborated this concept into the doctrine of "informed consent," requiring much more than mere acquiescence.

The essential operational elements of informed consent involve a careful assessment of the patient's decision-making capacity, the voluntariness of the decisions, and the nature and extent of the information to be disclosed. Decision-making capacity is reflected in the patient's ability to comprehend, communicate, and appreciate the consequences of available choices. Voluntariness refers to the absence of internal or extrinsic pressures that may coercively restrict patient options.[8] Considerable controversy and legal variability surround the required content of the information disclosure. Traditionally, and still the law in many states, prevailing professional practice patterns have been accepted as the legal reference standard for required disclosure. The modern view, in furtherance of patient autonomy, rejects this so-called "professional" standard in favor of a lay, objective, "reasonable person" standard that requires physicians to disclose those material facts concerning treatment alternatives and risks that a reasonable person would need in order to make an informed decision.[9]

The law recognizes several exceptions to the informed consent doctrine that may apply in cases involving CPR and life-support treatment. In emergency situations where the patient has lost decision-making capacity, consent may be implied. Where there is strong reason to believe that the disclosure involved may cause serious psychological harm, physicians may rely on a "therapeutic privilege" and be excused for failure to obtain informed consent.[10]

States vary considerably with respect to their statutory or common law definition of informed consent.[11]

III. The Parent–Child–Professional Triad

A. Parental vs. Children's Rights

Variables that carry the potential for conflict and liability are introduced into the patient–professional relationship when the patient is a minor under parental guardianship. Parental decision-making on behalf of children, particularly in the area of life support treatment, can provoke tension between parental rights and the rights of children, between parental rights and the duty of the professional to the pediatric patient, and between the interests of the decision-makers and those of the state.

As a general rule, the law protects the natural rights of parents to raise children free from unwarranted state interference, on the presumption that parents will act in the best interests of their children.[12] Accordingly, parents are allowed considerable latitude in medical decision-making on behalf of their children, even where the choice may result in some detriment to the child.[13,14] These parental rights are conditional on the fulfillment of their duty to provide necessary care for their minor children. In situations where parents have failed to provide their children with at least a minimum standard of medical care, the state may assert its interest in protecting the welfare of children by invoking child neglect statutes to override parental wishes. Courts will regularly uphold such interventions when parental refusals may have life-threatening consequences for their children, even when such decisions are genuinely motivated by strong family convictions.[15] When the consequences for the child are grave but not life-threatening, however, states have varied in their willingness to intervene, reflecting the continuing tension between the rights of individual children and family privacy.[16] Thus, courts have overruled parental refusal to consent to recommended cosmetic surgery for a severely deformed child[17] but upheld parental objections to a spinal fusion to correct their child's paralytic scoliosis.[13]

The ambivalence of courts in reacting to medically inappropriate parental decisions is further exemplified in cases where the treatment chosen is predictably ineffective, but not immediately life-threatening. Thus, in one case the court ordered conventional chemotherapy for a child suffering from leukemia over the objections of the parents who preferred metabolic and laetrile treatment,[18] while another court upheld a parental decision to treat their child with laetrile, reasoning that the parents fulfilled the legal requirement of providing minimum treatment necessary by demonstrating that some medical opinion exists supporting the use of laetrile.[19]

B. "Baby Doe" Cases

The widely publicized "Baby Doe" cases involve decisions by parents and physicians to withhold life-sustaining treatment from severely handicapped or critically ill newborns. The general ethical and legal concepts of physician–patient relationships, informed consent, rights of the incompetent, and conflict between family and the state are at issue in the Baby Doe context.

The President's Commission for the Study of Ethical Problems in Medicine and Biomedical and Behavioral Research identified significant problems in the decision-making process concerning neonates and offered an approach to a "best interest" analysis, including the use of ethics committees for ambiguous cases.[20] Congress has recently passed controversial legislation designed to restrict decisions to withhold treatment from neonates to cases in which 1) the infant is chronically and irreversibly comatose, 2) the provision of such treatment would merely prolong dying or not be effective in ameliorating or correcting all of the infant's life-threatening conditions, or otherwise be futile in terms of survival of the infant, or 3) the provision of such treatment would be virtually futile in terms of the survival of the infant, and the treatment itself under such circumstances would be inhumane. The Department of Health and Human Services has construed these provisions narrowly and specifically excluded any considerations of the potential "quality of life" of the affected infant.[21]

Difficult decisions about initiating cardiopulmonary resuscitation in Baby-Doe-like cases may arise unexpectedly in the delivery room with the birth of a very premature, critically ill neonate or baby with multiple congenital malformations. In general, estimates of ultimate survivability should be deferred and resuscitation attempted for all live-born neonates — in order to gain sufficient time for thorough diagnostic assessment and review of therapeutic options. In most cases, a well-documented review of

the clinical data supported by appropriate clinical consultation and discussions with family will result in a clear consensus concerning the appropriateness of continued life-support measures based on the child's best interest. Ethical dilemmas remain, however, in those complex cases where the participants in the decision-making process seek to balance the benefits of prolongation of life through the use of multiple invasive medical and surgical procedures against the burden of severely impaired quality of life for the child and family. The use of ethics committees as vehicles for ensuring careful consideration of the clinical and ethical issues in such cases has been widely endorsed.[20,22]

C. Consent of Minors

Historically, full rights of self-determination were available to children on reaching the legal age of maturity, defined as 18 years. Legislatures and courts have expanded minors' rights to give consent for medical treatment. A child may acquire status as an "emancipated minor" entitled to treatment as an adult by marriage, judicial decree, military service, parental consent, failure by the parents to meet legal responsibilities, living apart from and financially independent of parents and, in some circumstances, motherhood. In addition, statutory "mature minor" rules uphold the validity of consent given by minors over age 15, where the treatment is appropriate and the minor is considered capable of comprehending the clinical circumstances and therapeutic options.[23] However, implementation of the mature minor rule will often vary inversely with the gravity of the medical condition and the complexity of the proposed treatment.[24,25] Many state statutes permit minors to consent to treatment for specified conditions such as venereal disease and drug addiction. Some contemporary authorities propose a "variable competence" approach to minors' consent, taking into account developmental aspects of cognitive and psychosocial maturation.[26] As a child's powers to interpret and integrate life's experiences elaborates from a characteristically concrete, short-sighted perspective to an appreciation of abstract, future-oriented concepts, there may follow a concomitant expansion of decisional rights involving increasingly complex and risky alternatives. Professionals have been encouraged to obtain "assent" for some treatment from children as young as seven years and, in the interests of promoting childrens' rights, to pay due regard to persistent expressions of dissent by young children.[27]

It is not unreasonable to expect that, increasingly, situations will arise in which minors express a desire to participate in the decision-making process, including choices involving life-and-death consequences.[28]

IV. Essential Elements of Medical Malpractice

A. General Considerations

Medical malpractice actions are based on allegations of negligent conduct by the physician. To prevail, the patient must prove that the physician failed in his or her *duty* to provide *reasonably competent* care to that patient and that the *injury* complained of was *caused* by that failure. Each emphasized element of this definition must be supported separately by sufficient evidence to make the allegation more likely than not. Poor results, complications of treatment, errors in judgment are not necessarily evidence of malpractice.[4]

The physician's legal duty toward the patient begins with a prior mutual agreement to provide care for compensation or on any act that may represent an undertaking to provide care. The patient must prove that the physician breached that duty either by failing to provide care or by providing care that did not meet an acceptable standard. Further, the patient must, in fact, have suffered an injury. That is, despite evidence that the care provided was substandard, a claim of medical malpractice will fail if the patient was fortunate enough to escape injury. Finally, the plaintiff must prove that the physician's failure to provide care of an acceptable standard was the causative factor in the patient's injury.

While these elements apply generally to medical malpractice cases, specific criteria may vary considerably from state to state.

B. Standards of Care

1. General Standards

Key to the finding of medical malpractice is the *standard of care* by which the physician's conduct will be measured. Physicians are required to exercise that degree of care and skill expected of a reasonably competent practitioner of the same class, acting in the same or similar circumstances. Courts vary, however, about the geographic limits from which the comparison practitioner may be drawn. The traditional "strict locality rule," which limited the comparison standard to the same geographic area as the defendant physician, has been abandoned in many courts in favor of a regional or national standard.[29] Many courts, recognizing the widespread improvement in the standard of medical care, greater access to information and facilities, and standardized training programs for medical specialists, look to nationally accepted standards of care. As a practical matter, the use of a wider geographic standard expands considerably the range of medical expert opinions available to parties in malpractice litigation.

It is noteworthy that medical malpractice cases in cardiopulmonary resuscitation have been limited to in-hospital cases where the risk of cardiac arrest could be anticipated and that apparently no actions have been brought against volunteers attempting to rescue out-of-hospital cardiac arrest victims.[30] Moreover, Good Samaritan statutes, to be discussed further, have served to immunize potential rescuers from legal liability.

2. Standards for CPR

Determining the reference standard of care is often the key to medical malpractice litigation. A person at the scene of a cardiac arrest may be bound by a duty to provide care according to acceptable standards based on a prior relationship with the patient, such as that of the patient's attending physician, or by virtue of employment in an organized emergency medical services system, or by undertaking to assist the victim at the scene. The standard of care by which the rescuer's conduct may be measured in initiating, carrying out, or terminating cardiopulmonary resuscitation takes into account the class of the rescuer, the level of expertise that the rescuer may have or is expected to have, and the circumstances surrounding the event. Whether a person trained in CPR may be legally held to American Heart Association standards is unclear. Commentators have noted that some courts regard the American Heart Association CPR Guidelines as a national standard of care.[30,31]

C. Res Ipsa Loquitur

Under certain circumstances, a plaintiff may bring a successful medical malpractice action despite being unable to prove the presence of each of the previously described essential elements of negligence. The doctrine of *Res Ipsa Loquitur* ("the thing speaks for itself") allows a plaintiff to advance a medical malpractice claim by showing that the injury suffered does not ordinarily occur in the absence of negligence and that the instrumentality of the injury was in the exclusive control of the defendant.[32] The participation of many individuals in a resuscitation effort typically carried on in an atmosphere of confusion that may make collection of factual evidence difficult theoretically lends itself to this legal principle. However, the doctrine has been used infrequently in emergency care cases and is not permitted by the courts of many states in medical malpractice actions.[33] Moreover, given the odds against successful resuscitation in most circumstances, it is unlikely that a plaintiff could sustain a claim based on a presumption of negligence causing a poor outcome.[34]

D. Failure to Obtain Consent

A corollary of the modern, complex view of informed consent is the multi-tiered requirement of proof in malpractice cases based on failure to obtain consent. The plaintiff must prove that the physician failed to disclose all the material facts that a reasonable person would require in order to make an informed decision, that the patient's injury was caused by the physician's act, for which the patient granted uninformed permission, and that a reasonable person would have withheld consent had the material facts been disclosed.[9]

Consent may be implied in cardiac arrest cases, as it is in any emergency where circumstances preclude an opportunity for prior discussion with the patient or guardian.

Difficult problems may arise in emergency departments or on the street, when documents on the victim's person or statements by family members purport to represent the victim's refusal of CPR. Authorities encourage the exercise of medical judgment in such cases.[6,33]

V. Hospital Liability

The professional providing CPR will often be functioning within a larger organizational context. Emergency room staff, hospital-based cardiac arrest teams, hospital medical staff, trained technicians in an emergency medical services system, municipal fire fighters, and police personnel are all tied to complex lines of accountability through which legal liabilities may flow.

A hospital may be held liable not only for the organized services it provides but also for the individual acts of its employees. A hospital that represents itself as operating an emergency room has a duty to accept and treat all patients coming to its doors and to provide a properly equipped facility.[35] A hospital has a positive duty to maintain sufficient personnel properly trained in CPR, to provide appropriate equipment for CPR, to implement an alerting system within the hospital, and to monitor performance. This legal duty of hospitals to ensure organization of cardiopulmonary resuscitation services and competence of cardiac arrest teams in their employ has, in most jurisdictions, deprived hospital-based personnel from the legal immunity available to out-of-hospital rescuers.[34]

A. Vicarious Liability

Customary CPR practices emphasize prompt designation of a leader from among the responders to a cardiac arrest. Questions of potential special liability of the leader for the actions of others may be raised. A similar issue may arise in connection with the role of hospital-based medical personnel directing care via telecommunications with emergency medical services personnel acting in the field and the associated hospital liability for those acts.

A traditional legal view applied the "Captain of the Ship Doctrine" to such cases whereby a leader would be held vicariously liable for the malpractice of others in the group, depending on his or her level of control or right of control of their conduct. The modern legal trend, generally articulated with reference to surgical teams, recognizes the distinct areas of expertise contributed by each of the members and tend to hold each to a standard of his class and ultimately to his employer rather than shift liability to the team leader.[36] A legal analysis of vicarious liability in CPR cases may require balancing the degree of actual control of the team leader or medical director over participants against the extent of task specialization and separation of accountability attributable to each.

B. Hospital Corporate Liability

In recent years, courts have expanded the notion of hospital liability beyond responsibility for the facility to include the duty to ensure competent medical care for all patients.[37,38] By this doctrine, a hospital is considered an entity composed of both administration and medical staff, salaried and volunteer, each sharing joint responsibility for the development of standards and monitoring the quality of patient care. With the acceptance of national standards of pediatric CPR, it is likely that courts will recognize hospital corporate liability for the provision of appropriate cardiopulmonary resuscitation services for infants and children, including appropriately trained personnel, proper equipment, an organized system for responding to pediatric cardiopulmonary arrests, and continuous monitoring of performance.

VI. Duty to Rescue

A. Ethical and Legal Aspects

The American Heart Association stresses the crucial role of the first responder acting in advance of the arrival of an organized resuscitation team.[39] Immediate at-the-scene bystander resuscitation efforts correlate positively with successful outcome.[40] A major goal, therefore, is to train as many as possible to perform CPR. These efforts in the professional and lay communities appear to be well-received and imbue the participants with a sense of competence and motivation.[41]

Under the generally accepted moral principle of beneficence, the fundamental proscription against actively harming others is complemented by an affirmative duty to benefit others when in a position to do so.[42] Traditional Anglo-American law, however, rejects the legal enforcement of this moral obligation. Precedents in case law distinguish between an affirmative act, which if performed inappropriately may give rise to liability in rescue situations, and failure to act, which, however ignoble, may be above legal reproach.[4,43] The moral paradox may result in which a person making a well-intentioned, but incompetent, attempt to rescue another could be held legally liable for failing to meet a reasonable standard of care while the indifferent bystander would escape liability altogether.

Certain preexisting relationships may create legal duties to rescue in emergency situations. These duties may stem from contractual relationships as in the case of emergency room physicians, police, life guards, or emergency medical technicians. Special status relationships, such as parent–child, captain–passenger, employer–employee, may carry a general legal duty to rescue, if the effort can be made without danger to the rescuer.[44]

Physicians, when not functioning in an official, contractually based capacity, are subject to similar disparate moral and legal standards. While physicians' moral obligation to assist in emergencies is asserted in the professional code of ethics,[3] no legal duty to act has been imposed simply because they are physicians.[45]

B. Good Samaritan Statutes

Despite reluctance to assign legal liability for failure to act, courts have ruled that once any steps are initiated that, if terminated, would place the victim in a worse position or compromise the likelihood of assistance from others, the potential rescuer incurs a legal duty to perform appropriately.[4] This element of the law of rescue, coupled with the dramatic growth in medical malpractice litigation, created well-grounded fear that professionals would be hesitant to offer assistance and, ultimately, led to Good Samaritan immunity statues in all states.

Good Samaritan statutory language generally identifies a *protected class*, usually focusing on protection of health professionals in order to encourage response by trained individuals. In some states, statutes protect any person offering emergency assistance. As a general rule, legal immunity is granted only to persons rendering aid *gratuitously*. However, many state statutes creating organized emergency medical services protect trained professionals in the course of their official duties.

The *scope of immunity* granted varies considerably among the statutes. Common to all is the requirement that the rescuer show "good faith" belief that the situation called for the immediate action undertaken. Most statutes confer legal immunity for incompetent rescue attempts unless the actions were *grossly negligent*, meaning conduct that would be considered reckless, offensive, and shocking to most people. The *scene of the acts* covered by Good Samaritan statutes also varies. In some states, only actions at the site of the emergency incident are covered, while others include events during transport to a medical facility.[46] In some statutes, immunity is extended to persons responding to an emergency within a hospital, provided they have no preexisting duty to offer assistance. In contrast, other states have denied protection to these same persons, reasoning that members of a hospital staff are presumed to have sufficient expertise in emergency medical care.[46]

Interestingly, recent enactment of statutes in Vermont[47] and Minnesota[48] requiring persons to offer emergency assistance may herald a movement away from the common law rule against recognizing a general duty to rescue.[48,49]

Although universally adopted, it is questionable whether Good Samaritan statutes add any protection from legal liability not already afforded by common law principles. Traditional legal concepts hold persons offering assistance in an emergency to a "reasonable care" standard, taking into account all of the circumstances surrounding the incident and the level of skill of the individual. Thus, the common law formula considers the existence of an emergency in determining what degree of care is reasonable.[50] Moreover, there is little empirical evidence that Good Samaritan statutes have been effective in relieving anxiety of professionals about litigation and promoting emergency rescue behavior.[45] The constitutionality of Good Samaritan statutes has also been called into question in that they tend effectively to deprive victims of the right to legal recourse where injuries were suffered because of incompetent care.[51] Finally, it has been pointed out that the qualified immunity granted by Good Samaritan statutes does not preclude injured plaintiffs from filing suits, a practice which the wide variability and ambiguity among statutes may serve to encourage.[52]

The capability and willingness of first responders to apply CPR to pediatric victims is of ultimate importance, especially in view of the epidemiology of cardiac arrest in that age group. The predominance of underlying respiratory etiologies for pediatric cardiac arrest and the duration of hypoxia–ischemia to the brain consequent to delayed attempts at resuscitation are thought largely to account for the poor out-of-hospital success rate.[5] While children stand to gain substantially from widespread dissemination of CPR skills through organized educational programs, first responders should not be dissuaded from making reasonable attempts at CPR, regardless of their level of experience or training, out of fear of possible subsequent litigation. Whether under good Samaritan statutes or traditional common law principles, it is likely that CPR attempts in emergency situations will be viewed as reasonable even when provided by an inadequately trained rescuer, as long as there was a good faith belief that the possible benefits of the attempt outweighed the risk of harm due to the rescuer's incompetence.[51] No legal cases have been reported in which a layperson was successfully sued having reasonably performed CPR.[53]

VII. Decisions to Initiate and Terminate CPR Attempts

First responders at the scene of a cardiac arrest are encouraged to initiate full CPR measures in virtually all instances, without attempting to assess resuscitability. The unreliability of criteria for immediately determining death, with a few exceptions, supports the standard requiring the rescuer to give the victim the benefit of the doubt and initiate attempts at resuscitation.[54] Unreliable or unverifiable information about prior illness of the victim or about wishes previously expressed by the victim against CPR should not influence the exercise of medical judgment in emergency situations.

A decision to terminate CPR, based on nonresuscitability, is equivalent to a determination of death and must therefore be made by a physician. Nonphysicians are required to continue CPR to the limits of their physical endurance or until the care of the victim is transferred to another qualified, responsible person. Physicians are required to continue CPR as necessary until the victim is transferred to the care of other properly trained personnel or suffers a cardiac death as defined by cardiovascular unresponsiveness to acceptable resuscitative techniques.[54]

Some investigators have proposed guidelines for cessation of CPR efforts based on predictability of cardiac recovery following specified periods of apnea, pulselessness, and resuscitation efforts.[55] Empirical studies demonstrate considerable physician variability in the interpretation of clinical data used in support of decisions to continue or terminate CPR.[56] This variability in clinical practice, together with the complex ethical and psychological factors at work in individual cases, have led some commentators to prefer that no specific criteria be promulgated for ceasing CPR.[57]

VIII. Orders Not to Resuscitate

In marked contrast to earlier times when most people died at home in the comfort of familiar surroundings, an estimated 80% of all deaths now occur in hospitals.[20] Given the deeply embued institutional imperative to employ all available means to prevent death, it is not surprising that a large proportion of hospitalized patients die after one or more attempts at CPR.[58] Recognizing that attempts at resuscitation may not always promote patient well being, the National Conference Steering Committee stated "the purpose of cardiopulmonary resuscitation is the prevention of sudden, unexpected death." Cardiopulmonary resuscitation may not be indicated in certain situations such as terminal, irreversible illness when death is not unexpected or where prolonged cardiac arrest dictates the futility of resuscitation efforts. Resuscitation in these circumstances may represent a positive violation of an individual's right to die with dignity. When CPR is considered not to be indicated for hospital patients, it is appropriate to note this in the patient's chart.[59] While this statement legitimizes decisions not to resuscitate, it leaves open the question of how and by whom its essential terms are defined. Notwithstanding diverse philosophical views about the morality of withholding or withdrawing life-saving treatment, modern courts have championed the cause of individual patient autonomy.

A. Competent Patients

Consistent with the principle of self-determination, a competent patient's right to refuse CPR is virtually absolute.[60,61] Courts have limited the right of the competent patient to refuse life-saving treatment in only a few narrowly defined circumstances, such as the protection of dependent children.[62]

In everyday legal contexts, such as the assignment of property rights, defining "competence" is straightforward. Determination of competence in terms of "decision-making capacity in the health care process" is considerably more complex, yet critical to an analysis of resuscitation decisions. Patients may have decisional capacity for some medical alternatives, but not for others. A "sliding scale" approach to competence has been suggested by which standards for valid consent or refusal become more stringent as the consequences of the decision become more serious.[63] The degree to which a patient's competence level may be temporarily or permanently affected by pain, drugs, or mental state must also be assessed.[64] Once competence has been established, the patient, under the consent doctrine, has the right to refuse treatment, including life-saving measures, even if the decision seems foolish or irrational to others.

Studies suggest that, notwithstanding these legal principles, wide disparities in physician practices exist with respect to discussing resuscitation with competent patients.[65,66] Legal considerations aside, communicative behavior among practitioners, patients, and families on the subject of resuscitation appears to be influenced significantly by social and ethical values held by staff members and by differing views concerning the propriety of including competent patients in such discussions.[67-72]

Situations may arise where minors express the wish to have life support treatment withheld.[28] There may be a tendency to underestimate the capacity of some adolescent patients to deal with concepts of death, terminal illness, and its consequences.[27] Courts may find that emancipated minors can legally determine their resuscitation status based on their own individual desires.[73]

B. Incompetent Patients

It is likely that a patient newly diagnosed as terminally ill will be incompetent at the time the matter of resuscitation is first raised. In one study, only about half such patients were still conscious 14 days after their diagnosis.[20] The dilemma promoting the autonomy of incompetent patients who are hopelessly ill has recently received considerable attention.[74] Though at times confusing and contradictory, some general themes begin to emerge from a review of certain court rulings.

It has clearly been stated that physicians have no obligation to provide futile or useless treatment. Thus, an order not to resuscitate an irreversibly terminally ill patient for whom resuscitation would merely prolong the dying process may be appropriate.[75] Nevertheless, the subjective value judgments inherent in such terms as "hopeless," "irreversible," and "terminal" should be recognized, and open discussion among participants in the decision-making process should be encouraged.[76]

A second important principle asserts that the right of self-determination vested in competent patients is equally available to the incompetent.[77] Therefore, proxy decision-makers engaged in decisions about life-sustaining treatment or determining the appropriate resuscitation status for incompetent patients are required to ascertain and represent, to the extent possible, wishes expressed by the patient while still competent. In applying this "substituted judgment" standard, the surrogate attempts to reach the decision that the incapacitated person would make if he or she were able to choose. Previous written or oral statements or other indirect or trustworthy evidence of the patient's views regarding life-sustaining treatment or resuscitation will have weight as legal ground for substituted judgment by the surrogate decision-maker.[78] Where it is not possible to ascertain the patient's prior wishes or where the patient never was competent, as in the case of minors, physicians and surrogates may, in some jurisdictions, decide the resuscitation status based on their assessment of the patient's "best interests."[79]

Designations of treatments as "ordinary" or "extraordinary" have a long tradition of utility as features that distinguish obligatory from optional care in assessing the best interests of patients. Recent cases recognize the ambiguity of those terms and prefer to shift analysis from the type of treatment to the condition of the patient. By this formula, the proportionality between potential benefit to the patient and the burden of the proposed treatment is weighed.[79] For example, CPR might be considered disproportionately burdensome when it offers no reasonable possibility of more than very short term survival.

Physicians have customarily regarded next of kin as appropriate surrogate decision-makers for incompetent patients, even in the absence of legal guardianship status. At least one state, however, apparently requires judicial review of decisions to withhold CPR from incompetent patients who have left no evidence of previously expressed wishes.[80] Other courts have held that, given appropriate clinical consultation and good faith agreement among family members and the absence of specific state statutes to the contrary, no judicial approval is required.[79] Assessment of the incompetent patient's best interest, according to some courts, may take into account such factors as relief of suffering, the potential for preservation or restoration of function, the quality as well as the extent of life sustained, and the impact of the decision on those people closest to the patient.[79]

Because the issue of previously expressed wishes has little practical applicability to minors, parental decisions to withhold CPR or other life-sustaining treatment from their children will necessarily be measured by the "best interest" test. Nevertheless, the surrogates are expected

to exercise their judgment as to the child's best interest from the point of view of the child, that is, what the child might choose, were he or she competent.[81] The conflicts that may arise between legitimate parental rights of family privacy and the state's interest in protecting the welfare of children will center on differing perceptions of whether life-sustaining treatment or CPR serves the best interest of an individual child. Where decisions must be made on behalf of never-competent patients, some commentators urge that the automony of the family unit be upheld by giving substantial deference to family guardians' reasonable interpretation of patients' best interests from the perspective of their own beliefs and values.[82]

C. Policies and Guidelines

In an effort to ensure protection of patient's rights in circumstances where potential rescuers must act rapidly, often with limited personal knowledge of the patient, many hospitals have adopted formal policies governing orders not to resuscitate. Explicit policies serve to encourage prior deliberation, help ensure adherence to informed consent requirements, and promote the assignment of decision-making responsibilities to appropriate persons. Provisions suggested for incorporation into policies include requirements that "do not resuscitate" orders be written in the order sheet, accompanied by progress notes that explain the rationale for the decision and identify the participants in the decision-making process and guidelines for prior judicial review in specifically enumerated circumstances.[80] Orders not to resuscitate refer exclusively to the initiation of resuscitative measures in the event of cardiac arrest and are entirely compatible with administration of all other diagnostic and therapeutic modalities consistent with agreed upon treatment goals.

"Partial codes," in which advance limits are set on the extent of resuscitation efforts to be offered an individual patient, are not an uncommon practice.[83] Although generally rationalized as serving the patient's presumed best interest, incomplete resuscitation procedures may be ethically and legally questionable. The American Heart Association standards provide that CPR should be continued until cardiac death supervenes, defined as cardiovascular unresponsiveness to acceptable resuscitative techniques.[53] "Partial codes" may be unjustifiable because they deny the patient an acceptable test of resuscitability.[66,71,76] "Do not resuscitate" policies and forms used at some institutions provide opportunities to list specific associated life-support interventions that may or may not be incorporated into the limitation of treatment plan during the *prearrest* phase.

D. Ethics Committees

Legal writers, professional organizations, and government agencies have recently recommended that hospitals establish Ethics Committees for the purpose of encouraging more systematic and principled approaches to medical decision-making. The major functions generally envisioned for ethics committees are education, development of hospital policies and guidelines, and case review. It is anticipated that by creating a readily available forum for the airing of difficult ethical dilemmas, engaging the hospital political process in the consideration of policies and guidelines related to medical ethics issues, and offering nonbinding case consultative advice, the protection of patients' rights will be enhanced with a minimum need for recourse to judicial intervention.[84] Experience to date suggests that a multidisciplinary ethics committee can serve as an effective institutional resource, particularly in cases where life and death decisions for incompetent patients have been frustrated by ambiguity, communication breakdown, disagreement, or apparent conflict of interest.

One of the major stimuli for the development of hospital-based ethics committees has been the controversy surrounding the care of critically ill or seriously handicapped neonates. Many hospitals now have infant care review committees, which may be organized separately or function as part of the larger ethics committee. Although many of the administrative and legal aspects of hospital ethics committees are still being developed, such groups appear to be playing an increasing role in decisions involving life support treatment.[85,86]

IX. Emergency Medical Services

Recent government initiatives supporting the establishment of emergency medical services systems have significantly enhanced the delivery of emergency care to the scene of cardiac arrest victims. These are complex, integrated systems of care with multidimensional responsibilities that include appropriate maintenance of equipment, delineation of standards of care at various levels of training, on-site decisions to initiate or terminate CPR, shared clinical and legal responsibility between the Emergency Medical Technician (EMT) and central medical control, and the application of immunity statutes to professional EMTs, all of which are areas of potential litigation.

Specially trained technicians (EMTs, paramedics) working within such systems will generally be held to a standard of care commensurate with their level of training or certification. Most states require paramedics to pass the Department of Transportation course reflecting criteria established by the Task Force on EMTs of the National Academy of Sciences/National Research Council. Because EMTs essentially practice emergency medicine outside the hospital, their scope of practice relies on explicit protocols and close physician direction from remote hospital control sites.[87] EMTs are required to initiate resuscitation attempts in virtually all instances without attempting to determine nonviability[88] and to resolve any doubts as to patient viability in favor of the patient. They may terminate CPR only by order of a physician.[89] EMTs are therefore required to continue resuscitation efforts until effective spontaneous circulation and ventilation have been restored or care of the patient has been transferred to another qualified responsible person who continues the effort, a physician or physician-directed person assumes responsibility, or the rescuer is exhausted and unable to continue resuscitation.[90]

The EMT in the field is not at liberty to disregard or countermand an order given him by a physician.[91] Conflicts may arise at the scene when an EMT and a physician who may be less skilled in prehospital emergency care respond to a cardiac arrest. EMTs are advised to defer immediately to the responsible physician-director of the emergency medical service system for resolution of such conflicts.

Most statutes establishing EMS services provide legal immunity from malpractice liability for EMTs, provided their conduct was not grossly negligent or reckless. As previously noted, ethical and policy questions have been raised about the appropriateness of granting immunity to persons whose profession it is to render emergency care. The benefits of encouraging EMS personnel to act without fear of litigation must be weighed against the harm of restricting legal recourse for those injured by negligent resuscitation efforts performed during the course of the EMT's duty.

Training programs and transport protocols for the prehospital system of emergency care are primarily designed to respond to adult cardiac arrest victims. There is evidence to suggest that some systems fall short of providing optimal care for children.[92] Promulgation of specific guidelines for pediatric emergency care, including cardiopulmonary resuscitation, may serve to define a national standard to which all systems will be held.

X. Brain Death

Modern life support technology permits the maintenance of heart and lung function for extended periods of time in patients with no or minimal brain function and with no possibility for recovery. These developments challenge traditional legal, cultural, and religious concepts of death and point to the need for reliable policy for determining when no further treatment, including cardiopulmonary resuscitation, is indicated.[93] Many states have enacted "brain death" statutes with language recommended by major professional organizations, including lawyers, physicians, and legislators, in the Model Uniform Determination of Death Act. Brain death statutes generally provide that an individual is legally dead when it has been determined according to accepted medical standards that there has been either 1) irreversible cessation of circulation and respiratory function or 2) irreversible cessation of all functions of the entire brain including the brain stem.[94] Even in jurisdictions without brain death statutes, courts have accepted medical testimony determining death based on neurological criteria.[95]

Establishing a diagnosis of brain death with certainty in children may be difficult. Specific criteria for brain death developed for adults have not been validated in large series of children. Authoritative statements that may serve as useful working guidelines have recently been issued for adults and children of various age groups. [96,97] Diagnosis of death based on neurologic criteria should be approached with particular caution in circumstances where interpretation of clinical findings may be difficult, e.g., hypothermia, drowning, or involvement of neuromuscular blocking agents or barbiturates. [98,99]

Cardiopulmonary support systems may be withdrawn from brain dead patients without judicial review or fear of subsequent legal repercussions. In homicide cases, courts have consistently rejected the accused assailants' defense that the discontinuation of cardiorespiratory support from the brain dead victim was actually the superceding cause of death. [100] Similarly, courts have authorized the discontinuance of cardiorespiratory support systems for brain dead victims of child abuse without affecting the criminal charges against the alleged abuser. [101]

Extraordinary situations have occurred where cardiopulmonary resuscitation or continued life support of comatose or brain dead pregnant women were provided for the protection of a viable fetus. [102–104] Rapid advances in perinatology have brought into focus the potential conflicts between maternal and fetal rights, especially where the life of a viable fetus is at stake. It may be anticipated that these conflicts of interest will occasionally include the pregnant woman's right to refuse life-sustaining treatment. [105]

XI. Advance Directives ("Living Wills")

Though unlikely to arise in pediatric settings, the subject of advance directives issued by patients concerning their treatment in the event of later incompetence is an important development in the protection of patients' rights of self-determination. As of 1990, 40 states and Washington, DC, have enacted living will, durable power of attorney, or natural death acts by which a competent patient may prescribe binding limits to CPR and life-sustaining measures to be employed in the event of future decisional incapacity. [106] Advance directives may serve to provide surrogate decision-makers with important evidence of an incompetent patient's wishes, even in states without living will statutes. [75] While still the subject of considerable ethical and legal controversy, the greatest value of such legislation may be the impetus it provides for discussions between patients and practitioners about decisions to forego life-sustaining treatment.

XII. The Delivery Room

Resuscitation is more often required in the first few minutes of life than at any other subsequent period. [39] Modern obstetrics and perinatology have dramatically improved the standard of care expected in the delivery room. Professional organizations have promulgated national standards for the appropriate organization of skilled personnel and equipment to ensure delivery of acceptable resuscitation services to high-risk neonates. [107] These national guidelines recommend hospital policies requiring explicit procedures for identifying high-risk deliveries, anticipating the need for CPR by ensuring the presence in the delivery room of individuals skilled in neonatal resuscitation, and the development of contingency plans for multiple births and other unusual circumstances. This may have important implications for legal liability of obstetricians, anesthesiologists, nurses, and pediatricians in delivery room settings.

The improved ability to predict the need for neonatal resuscitation by widespread use of fetal monitoring, increased sophistication in neonatal resuscitation, and the general availability of regional referral centers combine to provide a potentially high legal standard of care. Birth-related problems, often needing delivery room resuscitation, are the largest single source of malpractice suits against pediatricians. [108]

Conclusions

What, then, must the student of Basic and Advanced Life Support know about the ethical and legal obligations that attend newly acquired life-saving skills, particularly with respect to pediatric subjects?

1. The underlying premise of a training module specifically dedicated to pediatric CPR asserts that children are different and that appropriate management regimens cannot safely be derived simply from scaled down adult versions.
2. To the extent that American Heart Association CPR guidelines are accepted as a legal standard of care, performance of trainees in cases involving childhood cardiopulmonary arrest victims will be judged against the content of the pediatric basic and advanced life support courses.
3. In addition to distinguishing clinical and technical aspects peculiar to pediatric patients, these standards will also imply an appreciation of the respective rights of parents and children, the limits of parental authority, and the role of the state in protecting the welfare of children.
4. It is the responsibility of the professional to recognize when the rights of parents and children may clash in pursuit of conflicting interests, especially in the process of making decisions to withhold CPR, and to

use available institutional and judicial resources to ensure that the best interests of the child are upheld.

5. Where there exists substantial doubt about the authority or reasonableness of guardian requests to withhold CPR, a prescription in favor of resuscitation should govern professional conduct until a resolution of conflict can be achieved.

6. Where potential rescuers are unsure of their pediatric skills, they should nevertheless undertake good faith efforts at resuscitation to the limit of their ability, relying on legal protection based on common law doctrines or Good Samaritan statutes.

References

1. Kouwenhoven WB, Jude JR, Knickerbocker GG: Closed-chest cardiac massage. *JAMA* 173:1064, 1960.
2. Veatch RM: *A Theory of Medical Ethics*. New York, Basic Books, 1981, p 25.
3. *Current Opinion of the Judicial Council of the American Medical Association*, 1984, p IX.
4. *Prosser and Keeton on the Law of Torts*, 5 ed. St. Paul, West, 1984, pp 186, 341, 375, 378, 382.
5. Wadlington W, Waltz JR, Dworkin RB: *Law and Medicine*, New York, Foundation Press, 1980, p 470.
6. Rozovsky FA: *Consent to Treatment, A Practical Guide*. Boston, Little Brown, 1984, p 31, 439.
7. Scholendorff v Society of New York Hospital, 211 NY 125 105NE 91 (1914).
8. President's Commission for the Study of Ethical Problems in Medicine and Biomedical and Behavioral Research: *Making Health Care Decisions*, 1982, p 55.
9. Canterbury v Spence, 464 F.2d772, 787 (1972).
10. Capron AM: Informed Consent in Catastrophic Disease Treatment and Research. 123 U PA L R 340, 387 (1974).
11. Andrews LB: Informed Consent Statutes and the Decision Making Process. 5 *J Legal Medicine* 163 (1984).
12. Wisconsin v Yoder, 406 US 205, 1972.
13. In Re Green, 307 A2d. 279 (1972).
14. In Re Seiferth, 127 NE2d820 (1955).
15. Prince v Massachusetts, 321US158 (1944).
16. Rothman DJ, Rothman SM: *A Conflict Over Children's Rights*. Hastings Center Rep, June 1980, p 7.
17. In Re Sampson, 278NE2d918 (1972).
18. Custody of a Minor, 393NE2d836 (1979).
19. In Re Hofbauer, 393NE2d1009 (1979).
20. *Deciding to Forego Life Sustaining Treatment*. President's Commission for the Study of Ethical Problems in Medicine and Biomedical and Behavioral Research. pp 16, 227, 251, n58, 142, 443.
21. Pub L 98-457; Fed Reg 45CFR part 1340; April 15, 1985, p 14878.
22. Wier R: *Selective Nontreatment of Handicapped Newborns*, Oxford University Press, 1984.
23. Capron AM: The competence of children as self-deciders in biomedical intervention, in Gaylin W, Macklin R (eds): *Who Speaks for the Child*. New York, Plenum, 1982, p 57.
24. Wadlington W: Minors and Health Care: The Age of Consent. 11 Osgood LJ, 115 (1973).
25. Bennett R: Allocation of Child Medical Care Decision Authority: A Suggested Interest Analysis. 62 Va L R 285 (1976).
26. Gaylin W: Competence, no longer all or nothing, in Gaylin W, Macklin R (eds): *Who Speaks for the Child*. New York, Plenum, 1982, p 57.
27. Leikin SL: Minors' assent or dissent to medical treatment. *J Pediatr* 102:169, 1983.
28. Schowalter J, Ferholt J, Mann N: The adolescent patient's decision to die. *Pediatrics* 51:97, 1973.
29. Shilkreit v The Annapolis Emergency Hospital Association 349A2d245 (1975).
30. *Proceedings of the First National Conference on the Medicolegal Implications of Emergency Medical Care*, American Heart Association, 1975, p 133, 155.
31. Dalen JE, Howe JT III, Membrino GE, McIntyre K: Sounding Board: CPR training for physicians. *New Eng J Med* 303:455, 1980.
32. Ibarra v Spangard 154P2d684 (1944).
33. Quimby CW Jr, Spies FK: Liability of the Hospital Cardiac Arrest Team 26 *Ark L R* 17, 24 (1972).
34. Mancini MR, Gale AT: Emergency Care and the Law, Aspen, MD, 1981, p 99.
35. Guerrero v Copper Queen Hospital 537P2d1329 (1975).
36. Sparger v Worley Hospital, Inc. 547SW2d582 (1977).
37. Darling v Charleston Community Memorial Hospital 211NE2d253 (1965).
38. Smith WB: Hospital liability for physician negligence. *JAMA* 251:447, 1984.
39. *Textbook of Advanced Cardiac Life Support*. American Heart Association, 1983, p 4, 241.
40. Cummins RO, Eisenberg MS: Prehospital cardiopulmonary resuscitation. Is it effective? *JAMA* 253:2408, 1985.
41. Anderson AM, Hoag, Sister B, Michelbach AP: Help When Needed. Lay Public Confident of CPR Skills *J Kans Med Soc* 81:572,1980.
42. Beauchamp TL, Childres TF: *Principles of Biomedical Ethics*, 2 ed. Oxford University NY 1983, p 148.
43. Weinrub EJ: The Case for a Duty to Rescue 90 *Yale L J* 247, 250 (1980).
44. Lipkin RJ: Beyond Good Samaritans and Moral Monsters: An Individualistic Justification of the General Legal Duty to Rescue 31 *UCLA L R* 252, 253, 262 (1983).
45. Helminski FJ: Good Samaritan Statutes: Time for Uniformity 27 *Wayne L R* 217, 221, 231 (1980).
46. Mapel FB III, Weigel CJ II: Good Samaritan Laws–Who Needs Them: The Current State of Good Samaritan Protection in the United States. 21 *So Tex L J* 327, 351 (1981).
47. VT Stat Ann tit 12, §519, (1973).
48. Minn Stat Ann, §605.05, (West 1983).
49. Feuerhelm KW: Taking Notice of Good Samaritan and Duty to Rescue Laws 11 *J Contemp Law* 219 (1984).
50. Restatement of Torts, Second 289, 296, 298 (1965).
51. Sullivan B: Some Thoughts on the Constitutionality of Good Samaritan Statutes 8 *Am J Law and Med* 27 (1982).
52. Norris JA: Current Status and Utility of Emergency Care Liability Laws, 15, *Forum* 377, 392, 402 (1980).
53. Standards and Guidelines for Cardiopulmonary Resuscitation (CPR) and Emergency Cardiac Care (ECC). *JAMA* 244:453, 505 1980.
54. Standards and Guidelines for Cardiopulmonary Resuscitation (CPR) and Emergency Cardiac Care (ECC). *JAMA* 255:2980, 1986.
55. Eliastam M, Duralde T, Martinez F, Schwartz D: Cardiac arrest in the emergency medical service system: Guidelines for resuscitation. *Ann Emerg Med* 6:525, 1979.
56. Eliastam M: When to stop cardiopulmonary resuscitation. *Topics Emerg Med* 1:109, 1979.
57. Chipman C, Adelman R, Sexton G: Criteria for cessation of CPR in the emergency department. *Ann Emerg Med* 10:11, 1981.
58. DeBard ML: Cardiopulmonary resuscitation: Analysis of six years' experience and review of the literature. *Ann Emerg Med* 10:408, 1981.
59. Standards for Cardiopulmonary Resuscitation (CPR) and Emergency Cardiac Care. *JAMA* 227(suppl): 864, 1974.
60. Satz v Perlmutter 362So2d160 (1978).
61. Lane v Candura 376NE2d1232 (1978).
62. Belchertown State School v Saikewicz 370NE2d417, 425 (1977).
63. Drane JF: The Many Faces of Competency. *Hastings Center Report*, April 1985, p 17.
64. Jackson DL, Youngner S: Patient autonomy and ''death with dignity:'' Some clinical caveats. *N Engl J Med* 301:404, 1979.
65. Bedell SE, Delbanco TL: Choices about cardiopulmonary resuscitation in the hospital: When do physicians talk with patients. *N Engl J Med* 310:1089, 1984.
66. Evans AL, Brody BA: The do-not-resuscitate order in teaching hospitals. *JAMA* 253:2236, 1985.
67. Eisenberg JM: Sociologic influences on decision-making by clinicians. *Ann Int Med* 90:957, 1979.
68. Youngner S, Jackson DL, Allen M: Staff attitudes towards the care of the critically ill in the medical intensive care unit. *Crit Care Med* 7:35, 1979.

69. Spencer SS: Sounding Board: "Code or no code:" A non-legal opinion. *N Engl J Med* 300:138, 1979.
70. McPhail A, Moore S, O'Connor J, Woodward C: One hospital's experience with a "do not resuscitate" policy. *Can Med Assoc J* 125:830, 1981.
71. Robertson J: *The Rights of the Critically Ill*. New York, Bantam, 1983, pp 77, 79, 100.
72. Farber NJ, Bowman SM, Major DA, Green WP: Cardiopulmonary resuscitation (CPR). Patient factors and decision making. *Arch Intern Med* 144:2229, 1984.
73. Hashimoto DM: A Structural Analysis of the Physician–Patient Relationship in No–Code Decision Making. 93 *Yale L J* 363, 381 (1983).
74. Wanzer SH, Adelstein SJ, Cranford RE, et al: The physician's responsibility toward hopelessly ill patients. *N Engl J Med* 310:955,1984.
75. In re Dinnerstein 380NE2d134 (1978).
76. Lo B, Steinbrook RL: Deciding whether to resuscitate. *Arch Intern Med* 143:1561, 1983.
77. In re Quinlan 355A2d647 (1976).
78. In re Conroy 486A2d1209 (1985).
79. Barber v Superior Court 195 Cal Rptr 484 (1983).
80. In re Storar 52NY2d363 (1981).
81. Custody of a Minor 434NE2d601 (1982).
82. Veatch RM: Limits of Guardian Treatment Refused: A Reasonableness Standard. 9 *Amer J Law and Med* 427 (1983–1984).
83. Younger SJ, Lewandowski W, McClish DK, Juknialis BW, Coulton C, Bartlett ET: "Do not resuscitate" orders — Incidence and implications in a medical intensive care unit. *JAMA* 253:54, 1985.
84. Cranford RE: Doudera AE: *Institutional Ethics Committees and Health Care Decision Making*. Ann Arbor, Health Adm, 1983.
85. Fost N, Cranford RE: Hospital ethics committees: Administrative aspects. *JAMA* 253:2687, 1985.
86. A.M.A. Judicial Council guidelines for ethics committees in health care institutions. *JAMA* 253:2698, 1985.
87. Smith JP, Boudai BI: The urban paramedic scope of practice. *JAMA* 253:544, 1985.
88. 5 *EMT Legal Bull* 4, 1981.
89. 7 *EMT Legal Bull* 7, 1983.
90. 5 *EMT Legal Bull* 3, 1981.
91. Caroline NL: *Emergency Care in the Streets*, 2 ed. Boston, Little Brown & Co. p 7, 1983.
92. Seidel JS, Hornbein M, Yoshiyama K, Kuznets D, Finkelstein JZ, St Geme JW Jr: Emergency medical services in the pediatric patient: Are needs being met? *Pediatrics* 73:769, 1984.
93. *Defining Death*. President's Commission for the Study of Ethical Problems in Medicine and Biomedical and Behavioral Research, 1981, p 13.
94. Guidelines for the determination of death. *JAMA* 246:2184, 1981.
95. Commonwealth v Golston 366NE2d744, 1977.
96. *Guidelines on the Termination of Life-Sustaining Treatment in the Care of the Dying: A Report by the Hastings Center*, Briarcliff Manor, New York, 1987, p 85.
97. Report of Special Task Force: Guidelines for the determination of brain death in children. *Pediatrics* 80:298, 1987.
98. Freeman JM, Rogers MC: On death, dying and decisions. *Pediatrics* 66:637, 1980.
99. Robinson RO: Brain death in children. *Arch J Dis Child* 56:657, 1981.
100. Eisner JM, Randell LL, Tilson JQ: Judicial decisions concerning brain death. *Conn Med* 46:193, 1982.
101. Cook JW, Hirsch L: *I: Medicine and Law.* 135, 140 (1982).
102. Dillon WP, Lee RV, Tronolone MJ, Buckwald S, Foote RJ: Life support and maternal brain death during pregnancy. *JAMA* 248:1089, 1982.
103. Siegler M: Brain death and live birth (editorial). *JAMA* 248:1101, 1982.
104. Veatch RM: Maternal brain death: An ethicist's thoughts. *JAMA* 248:1102, 1982.
105. Bowes WA Jr, Selgestad B: Fetal versus maternal rights: medical and legal perpectives. *Obstet Gynecol* 58:209, 1981.
106. Society for the Right to Die. September 1990.
107. *Guidelines for Perinatal Care*. American Academy of Pediatrics, American College of Obstetricians and Gynecologists, 1983.
108. *American Academy of Pediatrics News*. February 1985.

Appendices

Appendix A: Infant and Child Basic Life Support Sequence of Action Sheets for Cardiopulmonary Resuscitation and Foreign Body Airway Obstruction (FBAO) Management

Infant CPR
Infant FBAO Management: Conscious
Infant FBAO Management: Unconscious
Child One-Rescuer CPR
Child Two-Rescuer CPR
Child FBAO Management: Conscious
Child FBAO Management: Unconscious
Summary Sheets
    Cardiopulmonary Resuscitation (CPR)
    Foreign Body Airway Obstruction Management

Infant CPR

Step	Objective	Critical Performance
1. **A**IRWAY	Assessment: Determine unresponsiveness.	Tap or gently shake shoulder.
	Call for help.	Call out "Help!"
	Position the infant.	Turn on back as unit, supporting head and neck.
		Place on firm, hard surface.
	Open the airway.	Use head-tilt/chin-lift maneuver to sniffing or neutral position.
		Do not overextend the head.
2. **B**REATHING	Assessment: Determine breathlessness.	Maintain open airway.
		Ear over mouth, observe chest: look, listen, feel for breathing (3–5 sec).
	Ventilate twice.	Maintain open airway.
		Make tight seal on infant's mouth and nose with rescuer's mouth.
		Ventilate 2 times at 1–1.5 sec/inflation.
		Observe chest rise.
		Allow deflation between breaths.
3. **C**IRCULATION	Assessment: Determine pulselessness.	Feel for brachial pulse (5–10 sec).
		Maintain head-tilt with other hand.
	Activate EMS system.	If someone responded to call for help, send him/her to activate EMS system.
		Total time, Step 1—Activate EMS system: 15–35 sec.
	Begin chest compressions.	Imagine line between nipples (intermammary line).
		Place 2–3 fingers on sternum, 1 finger's width below intermammary line.
		Equal compression–relaxation.
		Compress vertically, ½ to 1 inches.
		Keep fingers on sternum during upstroke.
		Complete chest relaxation on upstroke.
		Say any helpful mnemonic.
		Compression rate: at least 100/min (5 in 3 sec or less).
4. Compression/Ventilation Cycles	Do 10 cycles of 5 compressions and 1 ventilation.	Proper compression/ventilation ratio: 5 compressions to 1 slow ventilation per cycle.
		Pause for ventilation.
		Observe chest rise: 1–1.5 sec/inflation; 10 cycles/45 sec or less.
5. Reassessment	Determine pulselessness.	Feel for brachial pulse (5 sec).* If there is no pulse, go to Step 6.
6. Continue CPR	Ventilate once.	Ventilate 1 time.
		Observe chest rise: 1–1.5 sec/inflation.
	Resume compression/ ventilation cycles.	Feel for brachial pulse every few minutes.

* If pulse is present, open airway and check for spontaneous breathing.
(a) If breathing is present, maintain open airway and monitor breathing and pulse. (b) If breathing is absent, perform rescue breathing at 20 times/min and monitor pulse.

Infant FBAO Management: Conscious*

Step	Objective	Critical Performance
1. Assessment	Determine airway obstruction.*	Observe breathing difficulties.*
2. Back Blows	Deliver 4 back blows.	Supporting head and neck with one hand, straddle infant face down, head lower than trunk, over your forearm supported on your thigh.
		Deliver 4 back blows, forcefully, between the shoulder blades with the heel of the hand (3–5 sec).
3. Chest Thrusts	Deliver 4 chest thrusts.	While supporting the head, sandwich infant between your hands and turn on back, with head lower than trunk.
		Deliver 4 thrusts in the midsternal region in the same manner as external chest compressions, but at a slower rate (3–5 sec).
4. Sequencing	Repeat sequence.	Repeat Steps 2 and 3 until either the foreign body is expelled or the infant becomes unconscious (see below).

Infant with Obstructed Airway Becomes Unconscious (Optional Testing Sequence)

Step	Objective	Critical Performance
5. Call for Help.	Call for help.	Call out "Help!" or, if others respond, activate EMS system.
6. Foreign Body Check	Manual removal of foreign body if one is found (tongue–jaw lift, NOT blind finger sweep).	Keep victim's face up.
		Place thumb in infant's mouth, over tongue. Lift tongue and jaw forward with fingers wrapped around lower jaw.
		Look into mouth; remove foreign body ONLY IF VISUALIZED.
7. Breathing Attempt	Ventilate.	Open airway with head-tilt/chin-lift.
		Seal mouth and nose properly.
		Attempt to ventilate.
8. Back Blows	(Airway is obstructed.) Deliver 4 back blows.	Supporting head and neck with one hand, straddle infant face down, head lower than trunk, over your forearm supported on your thigh.
		Deliver 4 back blows, forcefully, between the shoulder blades with the heel of the hand (3–5 sec).
9. Chest Thrusts	Deliver 4 chest thrusts.	While supporting the head and neck, sandwich infant between your hands and turn on back, with head lower than trunk.
		Deliver 4 thrusts in the midsternal region in the same manner as external chest compressions, but at a slower rate (3–5 sec).
10. Foreign Body Check	(Airway remains obstructed.) Manual removal of foreign body if one is found.	Keep victim's face up.
		Do tongue–jaw lift, but NOT blind finger sweep.
		Look into mouth, remove foreign body ONLY IF VISUALIZED.
11. Breathing Attempt	Ventilate.	Open airway with head-tilt/chin-lift.
		Seal mouth and nose properly.
		Reattempt to ventilate.
12. Sequencing	(Airway remains obstructed.) Repeat sequence.	Repeat Steps 8–11 until successful.†

* This procedure should be initiated in a conscious infant only if the airway obstruction is due to a witnessed or strongly suspected aspiration and if respiratory difficulty is increasing and the cough is ineffective. If the obstruction is caused by airway swelling due to infections, such as epiglottitis or croup, these procedures may be harmful; the infant should be rushed to the nearest ALS facility, allowing the infant to maintain the position of maximum comfort.

† After airway obstruction is cleared, ventilate twice and proceed with CPR as indicated.

Infant FBAO Management: Unconscious

Step	Objective	Critical Performance
1. Assessment	Determine unresponsiveness.	Tap or gently shake shoulder.
	Call for help.	Call out "Help!"
	Position the infant.	Turn on back as unit, if necessary, supporting head and neck.
		Place on firm, hard surface.
	Open the airway.	Use head-tilt/chin-lift maneuver to sniffing or neutral position.
		Do not overextend the head.
	Determine breathlessness.	Maintain open airway.
		Ear over mouth, observe chest: look, listen, feel for breathing (3–5 sec).
2. Breathing Attempt	Ventilate.	Maintain open airway.
		Make tight seal on mouth and nose of infant with rescuer's mouth.
		Attempt to ventilate.
	(Airway is obstructed.) Ventilate.	Reposition infant's head.
		Seal mouth and nose properly.
		Reattempt to ventilate.
	(Airway remains obstructed.) Activate EMS system	If someone responded to call for help, send him/her to activate EMS system.
3. Back Blows	Deliver 4 back blows.	Supporting head and neck with one hand, straddle infant face down, head lower than trunk, over your forearm supported on your thigh.
		Deliver 4 back blows, forcefully, between the shoulder blades with the heel of the hand (3–5 sec).
4. Chest Thrusts	Deliver 4 chest thrusts.	While supporting the head and neck, sandwich infant between your hands and turn on back, with head lower than trunk.
		Deliver 4 thrusts in the midsternal region in the same manner as external chest compressions, but at a slower rate (3–5 sec).
5. Foreign Body Check	(Airway remains obstructed.) Manual removal of foreign body if one is found (tongue–jaw lift, NOT blind finger sweep).	Keep victim's face up.
		Place thumb in infant's mouth, over tongue. Lift tongue and jaw forward with fingers wrapped around lower jaw.
		Look into mouth; remove foreign body ONLY IF VISUALIZED.
6. Breathing Attempt	Ventilate.	Open airway with head-tilt/chin-lift.
		Seal mouth and nose properly.
		Reattempt to ventilate.
7. Sequencing	Repeat sequence.	Repeat Steps 3–6 until successful.*

* After airway obstruction is cleared, ventilate twice and proceed with CPR as indicated.

Child One-Rescuer CPR*

Step	Objective	Critical Performance
1. AIRWAY	Assessment: Determine unresponsiveness.	Tap or gently shake shoulder.
		Shout "Are you OK?"
	Call for help.	Call out "Help!"
	Position the victim.	Turn on back as unit, if necessary, supporting head and neck (4–10 sec).
	Open the airway.	Use head-tilt/chin-lift maneuver.
2. BREATHING	Assessment: Determine breathlessness.	Maintain open airway.
		Ear over mouth, observe chest: look, listen, feel for breathing (3–5 sec).
	Ventilate twice.	Maintain open airway.
		Seal mouth and nose properly.
		Ventilate 2 times at 1–1.5 sec/inflation.
		Observe chest rise.
		Allow deflation between breaths.
3. CIRCULATION	Assessment: Determine pulselessness.	Feel for carotid pulse on near side of victim (5–10 sec).
		Maintain head-tilt with other hand.
	Activate EMS system.	If someone responded to call for help, send him/her to activate EMS system.
		Total time, Step 1—Activate EMS system: 15–35 sec.
	Begin chest compressions.	Rescuer kneels by victim's shoulders.
		Landmark check prior to initial hand placement.§
		Proper hand position throughout.
		Rescuer's shoulders over victim's sternum.
		Equal compression–relaxation.
		Compress 1 to 1½ inches.
		Keep hand on sternum during upstroke.
		Complete chest relaxation on upstroke.
		Say any helpful mnemonic.
		Compression rate: 80–100/min (5 per 3–4 sec).
4. Compression/Ventilation Cycles	Do 10 cycles of 5 compressions and 1 ventilation.	Proper compression/ventilation ratio: 5 compressions to 1 slow ventilation per cycle.
		Observe chest rise: 1–1.5 sec/inflation (10 cycles/60–87 sec).
5. Reassessment†	Determine pulselessness.	Feel for carotid pulse (5 sec).‡ If there is no pulse, go to Step 6.
6. Continue CPR	Ventilate once.	Ventilate one time.
		Observe chest rise: 1–1.5 sec/inflation.
	Resume compression/ventilation cycles	Feel for carotid pulse every few minutes.

* If child is above age of approximately 8 years, the method for adults should be used.

† 2nd rescuer arrives to replace 1st rescuer: (a) 2nd rescuer identifies self by saying "I know CPR. Can I help?" (b) 2nd rescuer then does pulse check in Step 5 and continues with Step 6. (During practice and testing only one rescuer actually ventilates the manikin. The 2nd rescuer simulates ventilation.) (c) 1st rescuer assesses the adequacy of 2nd rescuer's CPR by observing chest rise during ventilations and by checking the pulse during chest compressions.

‡ If pulse is present, open airway and check for spontaneous breathing. (a) If breathing is present, maintain open airway and monitor breathing and pulse. (b) If breathing is absent, perform rescue breathing at 15 times/min and monitor pulse.

§ Thereafter, check hand position visually.

Child Two-Rescuer CPR*

Step	Objective	Critical Performance
1. **A**IRWAY	**One rescuer (ventilator):**	
	Assessment: Determine unresponsiveness.	Tap or gently shake shoulder.
		Shout "Are you OK?"
	Position the victim.	Turn on back if necessary (4–10 sec).
	Open the airway.	Use a proper technique to open airway.
2. **B**REATHING	Assessment: Determine breathlessness.	Look, listen, and feel (3–5 sec).
	Ventilate twice.	Observe chest rise: 1–1.5 sec/inflation.
3. **C**IRCULATION	Assessment: Determine pulselessness.	Feel for carotid pulse (5–10 sec).
	State assessment results.	Say "No pulse."
	Other rescuer (compressor): Get into position for compressions.	Hand, shoulders in correct position.
	Locate landmark notch.	Landmark check.
4. Compression/Ventilation Cycles	**Compressor:** Begin chest compressions.	Correct ratio compressions/ventilations: 5/1.
		Compression rate: 80–100/min (5 compressions/3–4 sec).
		Say any helpful mnemonic.
		Stop compressing for each ventilation.
	Ventilator: Ventilate after every 5th compression and check compression effectiveness.	Ventilate 1 time (1–1.5 sec/inflation).
		Check pulse occasionally to assess compressions.
	(Minimum of 10 cycles.)	Time for 10 cycles: 40–53 sec.
5. Call for Switch	**Compressor:** Call for switch when fatigued.	Give clear signal to change.
		Compressor completes 5th compression.
		Ventilator completes ventilation after 5th compression.
6. Switch	Simultaneously switch:	
	Ventilator: Move to chest.	Move to chest.
		Become compressor.
		Get into position for compressions.
		Locate landmark notch.
	Compressor: Move to head.	Move to head.
		Become ventilator.
		Check carotid pulse (5 sec).
		Say "No pulse."
		Ventilate once (1–1.5 sec/inflation).†
7. Continue CPR	Resume compression/ventilation cycles.	Resume Step 4.

* (a) If CPR is in progress with one rescuer (layperson), the entrance of the two rescuers occurs after the completion of one rescuer's cycle of 5 compressions and 1 ventilation. The EMS should be activated first. The two new rescuers start with Step 6. (b) If CPR is in progress with one healthcare provider, the entrance of a second healthcare provider is at the end of a cycle after check for pulse by first rescuer. The new cycle starts with one ventilation by the first rescuer, and the second rescuer becomes the compressor.

† During practice and testing only one rescuer actually ventilates the manikin. The other rescuer simulates ventilation.

Child FBAO Management: Conscious*

Step	Objective	Critical Performance
1. Assessment	Determine airway obstruction.*	Ask "Are you choking?"
		Determine if victim can cough or speak.
2. Heimlich Maneuver	Perform abdominal thrusts (only if victim's cough is ineffective and there is increasing respiratory difficulty).	Stand behind the victim.
		Wrap arms around victim's waist.
		Make a fist with one hand and place the thumb side against victim's abdomen, in the midline slightly above the navel and well below the tip of the xiphoid.
		Grasp fist with the other hand.
		Press into the victim's abdomen with quick upward thrusts.
		Each thrust should be distinct and delivered with the intent of relieving the airway obstruction.
		Repeat thrusts until either the foreign body is expelled or the victim becomes unconscious (see below).

Victim with Obstructed Airway Becomes Unconscious (Optional Testing Sequence)

Step	Objective	Critical Performance
3. Positioning	Position the victim.	Turn on back as unit.
		Place face up, arms by side.
	Call for help.	Call out "Help!" or if others respond, activate EMS system.
4. Foreign Body Check	Manual removal of foreign body if one is found. DO NOT perform blind finger sweep.	Keep victim's face up.
		Use tongue–jaw lift to open mouth.
		Look into mouth; remove foreign body ONLY IF VISUALIZED.
5. Breathing Attempt	Ventilate.	Open airway with head-tilt/chin-lift.
		Seal mouth and nose properly.
		Attempt to ventilate.
6. Heimlich Maneuver	(Airway is obstructed.) Perform abdominal thrusts.	Kneel at victim's feet if on the floor, or stand at victim's feet if on a table.
		Place heel of one hand against victim's abdomen, in the midline slightly above navel and well below tip of xiphoid.
		Place second hand directly on top of first hand.
		Press into the abdomen with quick upward thrusts.
		Perform 6–10 abdominal thrusts.
7. Foreign Body Check	(Airway remains obstructed.) Manual removal of foreign body if one is found. DO NOT perform blind finger sweep.	Keep victim's face up.
		Use tongue–jaw lift to open mouth.
		Look into mouth; remove foreign body ONLY IF VISUALIZED.
8. Breathing Attempt	Ventilate.	Open airway with head-tilt/chin-lift.
		Seal mouth and nose properly.
		Reattempt to ventilate.
9. Sequencing	(Airway remains obstructed.) Repeat sequence.	Repeat Steps 6–8 until successful.†

* This procedure should be initiated in a conscious child only if the airway obstruction is due to a witnessed or strongly suspected aspiration and if respiratory difficulty is increasing and the cough is ineffective. If obstruction is caused by airway swelling due to infection such as epiglottitis or croup, these procedures may be harmful; the child should be rushed to the nearest ALS facility, allowing the child to maintain the position of maximum comfort.

† After airway obstruction is cleared, ventilate twice and proceed with CPR as indicated.

Child FBAO Management: Unconscious

Step	Objective	Critical Performance
1. Assessment	Determine unresponsiveness.	Tap or gently shake shoulder.
		Shout "Are you OK?"
	Call for help.	Call out "Help!"
	Position the victim.	Turn on back as unit, if necessary, supporting head and neck (4–10 sec).
	Open the airway.	Use head-tilt/chin-lift maneuver.
	Determine breathlessness.	Maintain open airway.
		Ear over mouth, observe chest: look, listen, feel for breathing (3–5 sec).
2. Breathing Attempt	Ventilate.	Maintain open airway.
		Seal mouth and nose properly.
		Attempt to ventilate.
	(Airway is obstructed.) Ventilate.	Reposition victim's head.
		Seal mouth and nose properly.
		Reattempt to ventilate.
	(Airway remains obstructed.) Activate EMS system.	If someone responded to call for help, send him/her to activate EMS system.
3. Heimlich Maneuver	Perform abdominal thrusts.	Kneel at victim's feet if on the floor, or stand at victim's feet if on a table.
		Place heel of one hand against victim's abdomen in the midline slightly above navel and well below tip of xiphoid.
		Place second hand directly on top of first hand.
		Press into the abdomen with quick upward thrusts.
		Each thrust should be distinct and delivered with the intent of relieving the airway.
		Perform 6–10 abdominal thrusts.
4. Foreign Body Check	(Airway remains obstructed.) Manual removal of foreign body if one is found. DO NOT perform blind finger sweep.	Keep victim's face up.
		Use tongue–jaw lift to open mouth.
		Look into mouth; remove foreign body ONLY IF VISUALIZED.
5. Breathing Attempt	Ventilate.	Open airway with head-tilt/chin-lift maneuver.
		Seal mouth and nose properly.
		Reattempt to ventilate.
6. Sequencing	Repeat sequence.	Repeat Steps 3–5 until successful.*

* After airway obstruction is cleared, ventilate twice and proceed with CPR as indicated.

BLS Summary Sheet
Cardiopulmonary Resuscitation (CPR)

	Objectives	Actions		
		Adult (over 8 yrs.)	**Child** (1 to 8 yrs.)	**Infant** (under 1 yr.)
A. Airway	1. Assessment: Determine unresponsiveness.	Tap or gently shake shoulder.		
		Say, "Are you okay?"		Observe
	2. Get help.	Call out "Help!"		
	3. Position the victim.	Turn on back as a unit, supporting head and neck if necessary. (4–10 seconds)		
	4. Open the airway.	Head-tilt/chin-lift		
B. Breathing	5. Assessment: Determine breathlessness.	Maintain open airway. Place ear over mouth, observing chest. Look, listen, feel for breathing. (3–5 seconds)		
	6. Give 2 rescue breaths.	Maintain open airway.		
		Seal mouth to mouth		mouth to nose/mouth
		Give 2 rescue breaths, 1 to 1½ seconds each. Observe chest rise. Allow lung deflation between breaths.		
	7. Option for obstructed airway	**a.** Reposition victim's head. Try again to give rescue breaths.		
		b. Activate the EMS system.		
		c. Give 6–10 subdiaphragmatic abdominal thrusts (the Heimlich maneuver).		Give 4 back blows.
				Give 4 chest thrusts.
		d. Tongue–jaw lift and finger sweep	Tongue–jaw lift, but finger sweep only if you see a foreign object.	
		If unsuccessful, repeat a, c, and d until successful.		
C. Circulation	8. Assessment: Determine pulselessness.	Feel for carotid pulse with one hand; maintain head-tilt with the other. (5–10 seconds)		Feel for brachial pulse; keep head-tilt.
	9. Activate EMS system.	If someone responded to call for help, send them to activate the EMS system.		
	Begin chest compressions: 10. Landmark check	Run middle finger along bottom edge of rib cage to notch at center (tip of sternum).		Imagine a line drawn between the nipples.
	11. Hand position	Place index finger next to finger on notch:		Place 2–3 fingers on sternum, 1 finger's width below line. Depress ½–1 in.
		Two hands next to index finger. Depress 1½–2 in.	Heel of one hand next to index finger. Depress 1–1½ in.	
	12. Compression rate	80–100 per minute		At least 100 per minute
CPR Cycles	13. Compressions to breaths.	2 breaths to every 15 compressions.	1 breath to every 5 compressions.	
	14. Number of cycles.	4 (52–73 seconds)	10 (60–87 seconds)	10 (45 seconds or less)
	15. Reassessment.	Feel for carotid pulse. (5 seconds)		Feel for brachial pulse.
		If no pulse, resume CPR, starting with 2 breaths.	If no pulse, resume CPR, starting with 1 breath.	
Option for entrance of 2nd rescuer: "I know CPR. Can I help?"	1st rescuer ends CPR.	End cycle with 2 rescue breaths.	End cycle with 1 rescue breath.	
	2nd rescuer checks pulse (5 seconds).	Feel for carotid pulse.		Feel for brachial pulse.
	If no pulse, 2nd rescuer begins CPR.	Begin one-rescuer CPR, starting with 2 breaths.	Begin one-rescuer CPR, starting with 1 breath.	
	1st rescuer monitors 2nd rescuer.	Watch for chest rise and fall during rescue breathing; check pulse during chest compressions.		
Option for pulse return	If no breathing, give rescue breaths.	1 breath every 5 seconds	1 breath every 4 seconds	1 breath every 3 seconds

BLS Summary Sheet
Foreign Body Airway Obstruction Management

	Objectives	Actions		
		Adult (over 8 yrs.)	**Child** (1 to 8 yrs.)	**Infant** (under 1 yr.)
Conscious Victim	1. Assessment: Determine airway obstruction.	Ask, "Are you choking?" Determine if victim can cough or speak.		Observe breathing difficulty.
	2. Act to relieve obstruction.	Perform subdiaphragmatic abdominal thrusts (Heimlich maneuver).		Give 4 back blows.
				Give 4 chest thrusts.
	Be persistent.	Repeat Step 2 until obstruction is relieved or victim becomes unconscious.		
Victim Who Becomes Unconscious	3. Position the victim; call for help.	Turn on back as a unit, supporting head and neck, face up, arms by sides. Call out, "Help!" If others come, activate EMS.		
	4. Check for foreign body.	Perform tongue–jaw lift and finger sweep.	Perform tongue–jaw lift. Remove foreign object only if you actually see it.	
	5. Give rescue breaths.	Open the airway with head-tilt/chin-lift. Try to give rescue breaths.		
	6. Act to relieve obstruction.	Perform subdiaphragmatic abdominal thrusts (Heimlich maneuver).		Give 4 back blows.
				Give 4 chest thrusts.
	7. Check for foreign body.	Perform tongue–jaw lift and finger sweep.	Perform tongue–jaw lift. Remove foreign object only if you actually see it.	
	8. Try again to give rescue breaths.	Open the airway with head-tilt/chin-lift. Try to give rescue breaths.		
	9. Be persistent.	Repeat Steps 6–8 until obstruction is relieved.		
Unconscious Victim	1. Assessment: Determine unresponsiveness.	Tap or gently shake shoulder. Shout, "Are you okay?"		Tap or gently shake shoulder.
	2. Call for help; position the victim.	Turn on back as a unit, supporting head and neck, face up, arms by sides. Call out, "Help!" If others come, activate EMS.		
	3. Open the airway.	Head-tilt/chin-lift		Head-tilt/chin-lift, but do not tilt too far.
	4. Assessment: Determine breathlessness	Maintain an open airway. Ear over mouth; observe chest. Look, listen, feel for breathing. (3–5 seconds)		
	5. Give rescue breaths.	Make mouth-to-mouth seal.		Make mouth-to-nose-and-mouth seal.
		Try to give rescue breaths.		
	6. Try again to give rescue breaths.	Reposition head. Try rescue breaths again.		
	7. Activate the EMS system.	If someone responded to the call for help, that person should activate the EMS system.		
	8. Act to relieve obstruction.	Perform subdiaphragmatic abdominal thrusts (Heimlich maneuver).		Give 4 back blows.
				Give 4 chest thrusts.
	9. Check for foreign body.	Perform tongue–jaw lift and finger sweep.	Perform tongue–jaw lift. Remove foreign object only if you actually see it.	
	10. Rescue breaths.	Open the airway with head-tilt/chin-lift. Try again to give rescue breaths.		
	11. Be persistent.	Repeat Steps 8–10 until obstruction is relieved.		

Appendix B: Medications, Equipment, and Records

Resuscitation Medications, by Weight and Age, for Infants and Children 0–10 Years

Age	50th Percentile Weight (kg)	Epinephrine		Atropine		Bicarbonate*	
		mg	mL	mg	mL	mEq	mL
Newborn	3.0	0.03	0.3	0.1	1.0	3.0	6.0
1 Month	4.0	0.04	0.4	0.1	1.0	4.0	8.0
3 Months	5.5	0.055	0.55	0.11	1.1	5.5	11.0
6 Months	7.0	0.07	0.7	0.14	1.4	7.0	7.0
1 Year	10.0	0.10	1.0	0.20	2.0	10.0	10.0
2 Years	12.0	0.12	1.2	0.24	2.4	12.0	12.0
3 Years	14.0	0.14	1.4	0.28	2.8	14.0	14.0
4 Years	16.0	0.16	1.6	0.32	3.2	16.0	16.0
5 Years	18.0	0.18	1.8	0.36	3.6	18.0	18.0
6 Years	20.0	0.20	2.0	0.40	4.0	20.0	20.0
7 Years	22.0	0.22	2.2	0.44	4.4	22.0	22.0
8 Years	25.0	0.25	2.5	0.50	5.0	25.0	25.0
9 Years	28.0	0.28	2.8	0.56	5.6	28.0	28.0
10 Years	34.0	0.34	3.4	0.68	6.8	34.0	34.0

Volume (mL) is based on the following concentrations:

    Epinephrine — 1:10,000 (0.1 mg/mL)

    Atropine — 0.1 mg/mL

    Bicarbonate — ≤ 3 months = 4.2% solution (0.5 mEq/mL)

                  > 3 months = 8.4% solution (1 mEq/mL)

*The use of bicarbonate in cardiac arrest is controversial (see text).

Good ventilation must be established before bicarbonate is used.

Infusion Medications, by Weight and Age, for Infants and Children 0–10 Years

ADD	0.6 mg (3 mL)* of **isoproterenol**
	0.6 mg (0.6 mL)* of **epinephrine**
	60.0 mg (1.5 mL)* of **dopamine**
	60.0 mg (2.4 mL)* of **dobutamine**

TO   100 mL of diluent

| INFUSE | at 1 mL/kg/hr or according to following table in order |

TO GIVE	0.1 µg/kg/min isoproterenol
	0.1 µg/kg/min epinephrine
	10 µg/kg/min dopamine
	10 µg/kg/min dobutamine

Age	50th Percentile Weight (kg)	Infusion Rate (mL/hr)
Newborn	3	3
1 Month	4	4
3 Months	5.5	5.5
6 Months	7.0	7.0
1 Year	10.0	10.0
2 Years	12.0	12.0
3 Years	14.0	14.0
4 Years	16.0	16.0
5 Years	18.0	18.0
6 Years	20.0	20.0
7 Years	22.0	22.0
8 Years	25.0	25.0
9 Years	28.0	28.0
10 Years	34.0	34.0

These are starting doses. Adjust concentration to dose and fluid tolerance.

*Based on the following concentrations: isoproterenol = 0.2 mg/mL
epinephrine = 1:1000 (1 mg/mL)
dopamine = 40 mg/mL
dobutamine = 25 mg/mL

Equipment Guidelines According to Age and Weight

Equipment	Age (50th Percentile Weight)					
	Premature Infant (1–2.5 kg)	Neonate (2.5–4.0 kg)	6 Months (7.0 kg)	1–2 Years (10–12 kg)	5 Years (16–18 kg)	8–10 Years (24–30 kg)
Airway — oral	infant (00)	infant/small (0)	small (1)	small (2)	medium (3)	medium/large (4/5)
Breathing						
Self-inflating bag	infant	infant	child	child	child	child/adult
O$_2$ ventilation mask	premature	newborn	infant/child	child	child	small adult
Endotracheal tube	2.5–3.0 (uncuffed)	3.0–3.5 (uncuffed)	3.5–4.0 (uncuffed)	4.0–4.5 (uncuffed)	5.0–5.5 (uncuffed)	5.5–6.5 (cuffed)
Laryngoscope blade	0 (straight)	1 (straight)	1 (straight)	1–2 (straight)	2 (straight or curved)	2–3 (straight or curved)
Suction/stylet (Fr)	6–8/6	8/6	8–10/6	10/6	14/14	14/14
Circulation						
BP cuff	newborn	newborn	infant	child	child	child/adult
Venous access						
Angiocath	22–24	22–24	22–24	20–22	18–20	16–20
Butterfly needle	25	23–25	23–25	23	20–23	18–21
Intracath	—	—	19	19	16	14
Arm board	6″	6″	6″–8″	8″	8″–15″	15″
Orogastric tube (Fr)	5	5–8	8	10	10–12	14–18
Chest tube (Fr)	10–14	12–18	14–20	14–24	20–32	28–38

Suggested Pediatric
Interhospital Referral Record

TO BE FILLED OUT BY REFERRING HOSPITAL   Date _____

Patient's name _____ Age _____ Sex _____ Weight (kg) _____

Parent's name _____ Parent's Phone _____

Patient's address _____

_____

Referring hospital _____ Phone _____

Referring physician _____ Phone _____

Receiving physician _____ Phone _____

MEDICAL INFORMATION (SEND COPY OF CHART)

Brief history _____

_____

_____

_____

_____

SERIAL ASSESSMENTS (SEE REVERSE SIDE; CHECK APPROPRIATE BOXES.)

For ventilated patient:

Endotracheal tube size	
Fi O_2	
Tidal volume	
Inspiratory time	
Peak inspiratory pressure	
Respiratory rate	
PEEP	

Arterial blood gas results

Initial _____

Latest _____

Intravenous lines: site(s) _____ fluid _____

Medications: _____

_____

_____

SERIAL ASSESSMENTS (Check the appropriate boxes or put the appropriate data in the boxes.)

Examination #	1	2	3	4	5	6
Time (AM/PM)	AM	AM	AM	AM	AM	AM
	PM	PM	PM	PM	PM	PM
Airway: Normal						
Intubated						
Breathing: Breaths per minute						
Work — Normal						
Increased						
Diminished						
Chest expansion: Normal						
Diminished						
Breath sounds: Normal						
Diminished						
Absent						
Circulation: Heart (beats per minute)						
Blood pressure (sys/diast)	/	/	/	/	/	/
Pulses — all absent						
Radial/pedal*	/	/	/	/	/	/
Femoral/brachial*	/	/	/	/	/	/
Perfusion: Capillary refill < 2 sec						
> 2 sec						
Toe temperature — Warm						
Cool						
Skin color — Pink						
Mottled						
Muscles — Normal						
Flaccid						
CNS: Recognizes parents/environment						
No recognition						
Withdraws from pain						
Posturing						
No response to pain						
Fluctuating level						
Pupils — Reactive						
Nonreactive						

* A = Absent; P = Present.

Appendix C: Overview of the Pediatric Advanced Life Support Course

The goals of the Pediatric Advanced Life Support Course are to provide the student with 1) information and strategies for preventing cardiopulmonary arrest in infants and children, 2) the information for recognizing the infant or child at risk of cardiopulmonary arrest, and 3) the cognitive and psychomotor skills necessary for resuscitating and stabilizing the infant or child victim of cardiopulmonary arrest. The course is intended for healthcare providers with responsibilities for the well-being of infants and children, i.e., pediatricians, housestaff, emergency physicians, family physicians, nurses, and paramedical personnel.

The 12¾-hour course is taught over 2 days, as outlined in "Course Timetable" later in this section. Lecture time is minimal so that hands-on experience can be emphasized. Technical skills and cognitive processes are first taught separately in small groups using 1-hour sessions. Practical application of these skills and knowledge in critical situations is then emphasized by using multiple case presentations. The case presentations occur in large group discussions called "integration sessions" and, subsequently, in small group teaching and evaluation stations.

The instructor's manual consists of seven sections, and this first section is an overview of the content and activities included in the course. The second section offers the instructor several teaching and learning strategies for effective instruction; the third is a detailed syllabus of course content, key teaching points, strategies for implementation in specific cases, and methods of evaluation; while the fourth presents details on the training of course instructors. Administrative considerations and responsibilities are covered in Section V, including planning checklists, flow diagrams, and evaluation forms for the completion of the course. Section VI provides supplemental course materials such as slide summaries, optional discussion questions, and student handouts; and Section VII outlines the faculty and course completion information that is specified by the American Heart Association.

The following summary is designed to provide the instructor with an overview, in the sequence recommended for teaching, of the content and activities presented in the *Textbook for Pediatric Advanced Life Support*.

Course Synopsis

Overview of Day 1

Lecture 1: Recognizing Respiratory Failure and Shock and Preventing Cardiopulmonary Arrest

This lecture will explore the antecedents of cardiopulmonary arrest. Signs and symptoms which suggest that a child is at risk will be presented. The student will be taught how to perform a rapid cardiopulmonary assessment. The central theme will be that if a child at high risk can be recognized, steps can be taken to prevent the arrest.

Skills Stations

The four skills stations are offered simultaneously and repeated so that each student will finish all four 60-minute stations in 4 hours.

Skills Station 1: Basic Life Support and Bag–Valve–Mask Ventilation: The steps in basic life support for the infant and the child will be demonstrated on a manikin, and the student will be given the opportunity to practice each step both separately and integrated into a resuscitation sequence. The theory behind each step will be reviewed. Bag–valve–mask ventilation will be discussed, demonstrated, and practiced.

Skills Station 2: Advanced Airway Management: Discussions will center on each piece of equipment and the indications for its use. Demonstrations and practice involve the use of airway adjuncts, endotracheal tubes, stylets, laryngoscopes/blades, large-bore suction catheters, and assistants to provide lip retraction and cricoid pressure. These techniques will be performed using manikin heads and anesthetized live animals, and each student will be given ample opportunity to practice.

Skills Station 3: Vascular Access, Fluids, and Medications: This skills station will teach a sequential approach to vascular access during resuscitation. Peripheral and central venous cannulation will be stressed, and the intraosseous technique will be presented as an alternative route for administering drugs and fluids. The pharmacology and use of resuscitation drugs and fluids will be discussed.

Skills Station 4: Rhythm Disturbances and Their Management: A simple approach to recognizing rhythm disturbances will be taught. Participants will practice identifying abnormal rhythms and their hemodynamic effects. The indications and methods for cardioversion and defibrillation for rhythm disturbances will be stressed, and drug therapy will also be presented.

Integration Session: Infant and Child Case Presentations

The integration sessions will give the students an opportunity to use the knowledge acquired from reading the text and participating in the skills stations to interact with the instructor in a case presentation format. In this session the priorities for airway management, resuscitation drugs, and defibrillation and cardioversion will be highlighted. In addition, priorities for resuscitation and the need for constant reevaluation after specific therapy will be discussed.

Lecture 2: Neonatal Resuscitation in the Emergency Room

In contrast to the delivery room, resuscitation of the neonate in the emergency department is often unexpected. This section will concentrate on the most important aspects of neonatal resuscitation, including airway management, warming, stimulation, suctioning, chest compressions, and the role of medication.

Overview of Day 2

Teaching Stations

The four teaching stations are given simultaneously and repeated so that the student will finish all four 45-minute teaching stations in 3 hours.

Teaching Station 1: Neonatal Resuscitation: The case format will be used to allow students, in small groups, to test their knowledge and psychomotor skills in the resuscitation of the neonate by responding to a scenario offered by the instructor. The basic principles of neonatal resuscitation will be stressed.

Teaching Stations 2, 3, and 4: Respiratory Failure, Shock, and Cardiopulmonary Arrest in the Infant and Child: These sessions will provide the participant with the opportunity to test his/her knowledge and psychomotor skills in the management of the pediatric patient in cardiopulmonary arrest, shock, or respiratory failure. Small groups of students will be expected to respond to a scenario given by the instructor and to demonstrate resuscitation using manikins, intubation heads, IV fluids, and drugs. The cases will be discussed with the group, and key teaching points will be highlighted.

Integration Session: Postresuscitation Stabilization and Transport

Cases will be presented that stress the principles of postresuscitation stabilization, airway and fluid management, and monitoring. Appropriate transport for ongoing care will also be discussed. Participants will be expected to respond to case scenarios in a format similar to the other integration session.

Evaluation Stations: 1. Neonatal Resuscitation; Cardiopulmonary Arrest in the Infant and Child. 2. Respiratory Failure in the Infant and Child; Shock in the Infant and Child. 3. Written Test

The three evaluation stations are given simultaneously and repeated so that each student will finish all three 45-minute stations in 2 hours, 15 minutes.

The evaluation stations will allow students, in small groups, to test their knowledge and psychomotor skills by responding to case scenarios offered by the instructor with the performance of resuscitation on a manikin using all appropriate techniques. The procedures and therapies will be recorded in the sequences they occurred, and each student will be critiqued on his/her performance.

The scenarios given will include cases of resuscitation of the newborn and respiratory failure, shock, and cardiopulmonary arrest in the infant and child.

The written test is an objective test designed to assess the student's knowledge of the materials given in the text as well as in the course. The participants will be asked to complete and turn in the course evaluation at the end of the test.

Panel Discussion

A brief panel discussion using the key faculty members will be held to give the students the opportunity to critique the techniques of the faculty and suggest additions to or deletions from the course materials.

Optional Drug Therapy Lecture

An optional drug lecture can be added to the course when the course director feels the audience would benefit from a more detailed discussion of drug therapy. An appropriate place for this lecture is after the skills station and before the newborn resuscitation lecture (Day 1).

Course Timetable

Day 1

Introduction	15 minutes
Lecture 1: Recognizing Respiratory Failure and Shock and Preventing Cardiopulmonary Arrest	45 minutes

Skills Stations:

1. Basic Life Support and Bag–Valve–Mask Ventilation	60 minutes
2. Advanced Airway Management	60 minutes
3. Vascular Access, Fluids, and Medications	60 minutes
4. Rhythm Disturbances and Their Management	60 minutes
Integration Session: Infant and Child Case Presentations	45 minutes
Optional Drug Therapy Lecture	30 minutes
Lecture 2: Neonatal Resuscitation in the Emergency Room	30 minutes

[Total teaching time: 6 hours, 15 minutes]

Day 2

Teaching Stations:

1. Neonatal Resuscitation	45 minutes
2. Respiratory Failure in the Infant and Child	45 minutes
3. Shock in the Infant and Child	45 minutes
4. Cardiopulmonary Arrest in the Infant and Child	45 minutes
Integration Session: Postresuscitation Stabilization and Transport	45 minutes

Evaluation Stations:

1. Neonatal Resuscitation; Cardiopulmonary Arrest in the Infant and Child	45 minutes
2. Respiratory Failure in the Infant and Child; Shock in the Infant and Child	45 minutes
3. Written Test	45 minutes
Panel: Summary, Questions, and Answers	30 minutes

[Total teaching time: 6 hours, 30 minutes]

Drug Delivery

Drug therapy in pediatric advanced life support has been simplified in the current recommendations of the American Heart Association.[1] Before discussing specific drug therapy, drug administration will be reviewed.

During a cardiac arrest, drug delivery is impaired. Because most drugs exert their actions on the central and arterial circulations, the drug must be transported from the site of administration through the right heart to the lungs and then back to the heart before it can be delivered to the arterial vascular bed. Central venous administration will therefore maximize drug delivery but is not always possible. To help flush the drug into the central circulation, a bolus of saline (2–5 mL) should be given after the resuscitation drug.

The intravenous and intraosseous routes are the preferred methods for drug administration during cardiopulmonary arrest. When vascular or intraosseous access is not readily available, initial resuscitation drugs may be given via the endotracheal route. Drug absorption after endotracheal administration depends on drug delivery to the distal small airways and alveoli.[2,3] Delivery of the drug can be facilitated by dilution with normal saline and administration through a catheter that extends beyond the end of the endotracheal tube. The use of a feeding tube or catheter may not always be practical, however, so diluted drugs can be instilled directly into the endotracheal tube and followed with 1–2 mL of saline to help distribute the drug into the lower airways. This should then be followed with several deep positive pressure breaths.

There are data showing that larger doses of resuscitation medications than normally given intravenously should be given when the endotracheal route is used.[4,5] Therefore, 0.2–0.3 mL/kg of 1:10,000 epinephrine (twofold to threefold the current recommended intravenous dose) should be used.

Drug Therapy Based on Cardiac Rhythm and Etiology of Arrest

Bradycardic rhythms are the second most common type of arrest-associated rhythms seen in the pediatric patient. Management is based on the underlying cause of the bradycardia. When it is associated with cardiac arrest (i.e., due to a severe hypoxic-ischemic insult), the resulting rhythm is often wide complex and not preceded by identifiable P waves. Patients with structural cardiac disease may develop bradycardia due to heart block or sinus node dysfunction. The therapeutic approach to patients

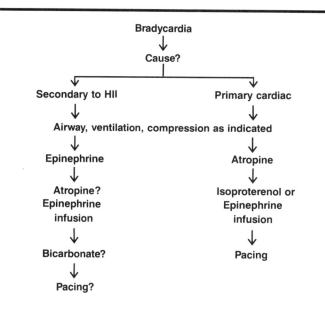

HII = hypoxic-ischemic insult

Figure 1

with primary cardiac causes of bradycardia differs from that of hypoxia-ischemia–induced bradycardia. Figure 1 outlines the approach to the treatment of bradycardia. Note that intubation, ventilation, and oxygenation **always** precede drug therapy.

Epinephrine (0.01 mg/kg [0.1 mL/kg] of a 1:10,000 solution) remains the drug of choice in hypoxia-ischemia–induced bradycardia. It is not likely that atropine would be helpful in this setting. If bolus administration of epinephrine is only transiently effective in postarrest bradycardia, a continuous chronotrope infusion is needed. Epinephrine infusion is preferable to isoproterenol because the latter often compromises coronary perfusion pressure, whereas epinephrine will maintain coronary blood flow.[6,7]

Although not common, primary cardiac disease must also be considered as a cause of symptomatic bradycardia. In this setting, **atropine** (0.02 mg/kg; minimum dose, 0.1 mg) may help accelerate the pacemaker rate. **Isoproterenol** and **epinephrine** infusions may also be effective therapy in this setting. Both epinephrine and isoproterenol infusions are administered in a dosage range of 0.05–1.0 µg/kg/min. Details on the preparation of these infusions may be found in chapter 5 (pages 55–58).

Cardiac pacing can also be helpful in primary cardiac bradycardia. This can be rapidly accomplished by external (transcutaneous), transvenous, or esophageal pacing. Pacing of the postarrest patient is rarely successful. Even if the electrical capture of the heart is achieved, pacing does not improve contractility and myocardial blood flow.

The administration of **sodium bicarbonate** may be considered for the patient who fails to respond to the therapy outline above or whose response is suboptimal due to severe acidosis. The limitations of bicarbonate administration are outlined in the section on asystole.

Asystole is the most common pediatric arrest rhythm. The management of asystole is outlined in Figure 2.

As shown in the figure, epinephrine is the drug of choice in asystole; there are no data showing that any other drug is effective. Basic life support with optimal ventilation, oxygenation, and perfusion (chest compressions) is essential and always precedes drug administration.

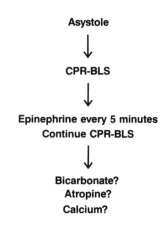

Asystole

↓

CPR-BLS

↓

Epinephrine every 5 minutes
Continue CPR-BLS

↓

Bicarbonate?
Atropine?
Calcium?

CPR = cardiopulmonary resuscitation
BLS = basic life support

Figure 2

Epinephrine is given in a dose of 0.01 mg/kg (0.1 mL/kg i.v. of 1:10,000 solution or 0.2–0.3 mL/kg via the endotracheal route). If this dose is not effective after 5 minutes, give at least twice the initial dose. This recommendation is based on data that show that the currently recommended dose is suboptimal and that larger doses are more effective in experimental models.[4,8] In addition, clinical data indicate that patients who do not have restoration of organized spontaneous cardiac activity after two rounds of epinephrine do not survive to leave the hospital.[9] Thus, giving a larger second dose to help restart the heart outweighs any potential risk from the use of larger drug doses.

Although no longer a first-line drug, **sodium bicarbonate** may be given if the patient is being adequately ventilated and the initial doses of epinephrine are not effective.

Bicarbonate will be effective only if the patient is being ventilated, oxygenated, and perfused. Remember to flush the intravenous line with normal saline after bicarbonate administration. The dose of bicarbonate is 1 mEq/kg.

There is no evidence that either atropine or calcium is useful in asystolic arrest. Therefore if they are used, neither should be given in preference to epinephrine. Calcium should be used only to treat documented hypocalcemia or to reverse the effects of hyperkalemia and hypermagnesemia.

Electromechanical dissociation (EMD) is a clinical state characterized by organized cardiac activity but absent pulses. EMD is most often seen as wide complex bradycardia in the postarrest setting. Drug therapy is the same as for asystole (i.e., epinephrine is the drug of choice), with an important caveat. The three correctable causes of EMD should always be considered: hypovolemia, tension pneumothorax, and pericardial tamponade. When EMD is caused by hypovolemia, then a narrow complex tachycardia or normal heart rate rather than a wide complex bradycardia is usually seen. Tension pneumothorax and pericardial tamponade also produce narrow complex rhythms, particularly in the early phases of these conditions.

Ventricular fibrillation and pulseless ventricular tachycardia are uncommon pediatric rhythms. Electrical defibrillation (2 J/kg; maximum first dose, 200 J) is the treatment of choice for these rhythms. The energy dose may be doubled if the first defibrillation attempt is unsuccessful (see Figure 3).

If defibrillation is unsuccessful, **epinephrine** is used in the management of ventricular fibrillation for the same reason it is useful in asystole—it increases coronary perfusion pressure and, therefore, myocardial blood flow. This helps restore myocardial cellular function and makes the heart more responsive to defibrillation. Epinephrine should be repeated every 5 minutes as required with subsequent larger doses (see the section on asystole).

Lidocaine is helpful in preventing the recurrence of ventricular fibrillation, but its administration should not delay defibrillation. Lidocaine is administered in a dose of 1 mg/kg after defibrillation. A second dose of 1 mg/kg may be given after 10–15 minutes. An infusion (20–50 µg/kg/min) should be started if the patient has structural heart disease, multiple premature ventricular contractions, or recurrent ventricular fibrillation. Instructions regarding the preparation of lidocaine drips are in chapter 5 (page 57). If the patient does not respond to defibrillation, epinephrine or lidocaine, **bretylium** should be used. The initial dose of bretylium is 5 mg/kg infused rapidly. The dose may be doubled if a second dose is required.

It is important to consider the other correctable causes of ventricular fibrillation and tachycardia, which include metabolic abnormalities (e.g., hyperkalemia), drug intoxication (e.g., tricyclics), and hypothermia.

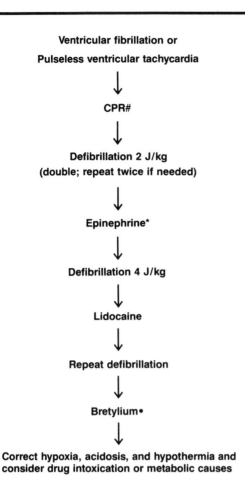

Ventricular fibrillation or
Pulseless ventricular tachycardia

↓

CPR#

↓

Defibrillation 2 J/kg
(double; repeat twice if needed)

↓

Epinephrine*

↓

Defibrillation 4 J/kg

↓

Lidocaine

↓

Repeat defibrillation

↓

Bretylium•

↓

Correct hypoxia, acidosis, and hypothermia and
consider drug intoxication or metabolic causes

NOTE—assess pulse after each intervention.

* Repeat epinephrine every 5 minutes of continued arrest.

• If needed, double dose to 10 mg/kg and repeat.

Figure 3

Postarrest Drug Therapy

The choice of drugs in the postarrest setting should be individualized for the patient, but there is no consensus for drug selection. It is important to keep in mind the goals of the initial therapy—restoration of adequate blood pressure and effective perfusion and correction of hypoxia and acidosis. These goals are vital to neurological preservation after an hypoxic-ischemic insult. Therefore, use the most potent drugs initially to stabilize the patient. If the patient improves, less potent agents can be substituted. Figure 4 summarizes this approach to stabilization of the postarrest patient in cardiogenic shock.

Postarrest patients are often poorly perfused, hypotensive, and acidotic. After a cardiac arrest, the most common reason for poor perfusion is cardiogenic shock; this is the result of arrest-associated myocardial ischemia. Some patients may also have poor lung compliance, which makes positive pressure ventilation difficult. In all patients, attention to ventilation, oxygenation, and perfusion are the initial steps.

Treatment of poor tissue perfusion is determined by the patient's hemodynamic state. In all patients, administration of a 10–20 mL/kg fluid bolus over several minutes is reasonable.

There are three inotropic agents used in the postarrest setting—dopamine, dobutamine, and epinephrine. Although in adults dopamine is often the drug of choice, in pediatric patients epinephrine is the drug of choice.

Epinephrine is a more potent vasoconstrictive agent and effectively increases myocardial perfusion pressure. The infusion rate of epinephrine varies between 0.05 and 1.0 μg/kg/min. Remember that a higher initial dose may be required in the hypotensive patient.

Dobutamine may be effective as a selective inotropic agent in the patient with poor perfusion and normal blood pressure. In children with cardiogenic shock, dobutamine increases cardiac output, decreases pulmonary wedge pressure (occlusive), and decreases systemic vascular resistance.[10] The dose is 5–20 μg/kg/min.

Dopamine may not be a very good inotropic agent in patients with poor myocardial function.[11] The advantage of this drug when used at low doses is its selective effect on renal and splanchic perfusion.

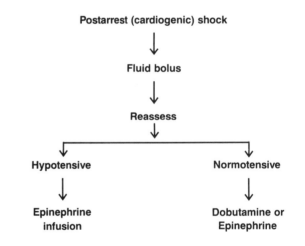

Postarrest (cardiogenic) shock

↓

Fluid bolus

↓

Reassess

↓

Hypotensive   Normotensive

↓   ↓

Epinephrine   Dobutamine or
infusion   Epinephrine

Figure 4

Selection of Inotropes in Nonarrest Setting

This summary of inotrope selection outlines an aggressive approach aimed at rapid initial stabilization. Therapy is determined by the type of shock.

Septic shock is characterized by a loss of peripheral vascular resistance, producing a wide pulse pressure due to the fall of diastolic blood pressure.[12] Hypotension usually occurs when the patient develops excessive vasodilation and leaking of fluid out of the vascular space. Hypotension may also result from poor cardiac contractility.[13]

Hemodynamically unstable patients are initially managed by aggressive fluid resuscitation. If there is no improvement in perfusion and blood pressure, use inotropic and vasoactive drugs. A drug that increases peripheral vascular tone is desired. If the patient is not hypotensive (i.e., in decompensated shock), a less potent vasoactive agent may be used. This approach is summarized in Figure 5.

It is important to recognize that the hypotensive septic patient may not respond to alpha-adrenergic vasoconstrictive agents in a normal manner.[14] Therefore, doses of infusion drugs may need to be high (as much as 1.0–1.5 μg/kg/min epinephrine or norepinephrine). Renal perfusion at these high doses will most likely not be compromised. On the contrary, if these drugs normalize the patient's blood pressure, renal perfusion should improve.[15] Both epinephrine and norepinephrine are potentially toxic agents but may be the only effective agents in the decompensated septic patient.

Norepinephrine is effective in the treatment of septic adults and may also be effective in pediatric patients for whom other measures have failed.[16]

Dopamine is a less potent peripheral vasoconstrictive agent and is helpful in less severely ill patients with sep-

sis. The initial starting infusion rate is 5–10 μg/kg/min. If infusion rates in excess of 20 μg/kg/min are required, the use of a more potent agent (i.e., epinephrine or norepinephrine) is indicated.

Reserve the use of **dobutamine** for patients with normal pressure and cardiac failure in which a selective inotrope is needed. Some patients with sepsis have significant myocardial dysfunction that produces cardiogenic shock.[13,17] Inadequate cardiac contractility can be recognized by the presence of decreased pulmonary compliance or overt pulmonary edema. Initial infusion rates are 5–10 μg/kg/min; rates in excess of 20 μg/kg/min suggest the need for a more potent agent.

Patients with **cardiogenic shock** are typically very poorly perfused, hypotensive, and very acidotic. Dobutamine is the drug of choice in the normotensive patient, whereas the more potent inotrope, epinephrine, is indicated in the hypotensive cardiogenic shock patient. Restoration of normal blood pressure with a potent vasoactive inotrope is important because coronary perfusion is dependent on an adequate perfusion pressure. Once pressure is restored, it is desirable to use a less potent vasoactive agent (e.g., dobutamine or dopamine) to avoid excessive afterload on the ventricle.

Hypovolemic shock should not be treated with inotropic agents; fluid resuscitation is the treatment of choice.

Caveats of Drug Infusion Therapy

When infusing any of the inotropic and vasoactive agents discussed above, remember that at the usual infusion rates, the drug may take 20 or more minutes to reach the patient, depending on where it is connected to the intravenous line. *Therefore, initially run the drip at fivefold to tenfold the initial rate* while carefully monitoring the heart rate and blood pressure. As soon as the heart rate begins to increase, decrease the drip rate to the desired infusion dose. The rapid clearance of these drugs prevents drug toxicity from the higher infusion rates as long as the rate is readjusted when drug effect is first seen. An alternative approach is to "Y"-connect the vasoactive infusion with an intravenous infusion flowing at a faster rate so that the vasoactive infusion is more rapidly carried to the patient. If this method is used, constant monitoring is required because sudden boluses of potent drugs may be rapidly delivered to the patient.

If you use the "Rule of 6" to calculate infusions, recognize that this rule does not work as well for heavier (> 20 kg) patients. The Rule of 6 is illustrated in Table 1. Note that other vasoactive drug infusions, although not discussed in this course, can be calculated with this same rule.

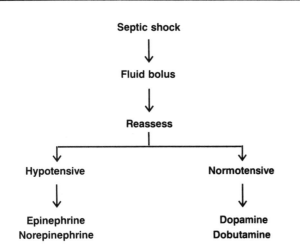

Figure 5

Table 1

Drug	Calculation Rule
Epinephrine	0.6 X body wt (kg)
Norepinephrine	= # mg to add to
Isoproterenol	diluent to make
Prostaglandin E_1	100 mL volume

Therefore, 1 mL/hr delivers 0.1 µg/kg/min.

Drug	Calculation Rule
Dopamine	6 × body wt (kg)
Dobutamine	= # mg to add to
Nitroprusside	diluent to make
Nitroglycerin	100 mL volume

Therefore, 1 mL/hr delivers 1 µg/kg/min.

For epinephrine, norepinephrine and isoproterenol, the calculation requires a large amount of drug when used in the heavier patient. This can easily be adjusted, however, by making an appropriate dilution. Thus, in a 20-kg child, the formula calls for 12 mg epinephrine (12 1-mL vials!). If a 1/10 dilution is made, then adding 1.2 mg to make a final volume of 100 mL makes a solution so that *10 mL/hr* delivers 0.1 µg/kg/min. The higher infusion rates are not a problem for heavier patients.

The Rule of 6 is also helpful to calculate infusions of prostaglandin E_1 (calculated like epinephrine) and nitroprusside and nitroglycerin (calculated like dopamine). Because these are not usual resuscitation drugs, refer to standard critical care textbooks for information on indications for use of these drugs.

References

1. Standards and guidelines for cardiopulmonary resuscitation (CPR) and emergency cardiac care (ECC). *JAMA* 1986;255:2841

2. Ward JT Jr: Endotracheal drug therapy. *Am J Emerg Med* 1983;1:71–82

3. Mace SE: Effect of technique of administration on plasma lidocaine levels. *Ann Emerg Med* 1986;15:552–556

4. Ralston SH, Tacker WA, Showen L, Carter A, Babbs CF: Endotracheal versus intravenous epinephrine during electromechanical dissociation with CPR in dogs. *Ann Emerg Med* 1985;14:1044–1048

5. Roberts JR, Greenberg MI, Knaub MA, Kendrick ZV, Baskin SI: Blood levels following intravenous and endotracheal epinephrine administration. *JACEP* 1979;8:53–56

6. Mueller H, Ayres SM, Gregory JJ, Giannelli S Jr, Grace WJ: Hemodynamics, coronary blood flow, and myocardial metabolism in coronary shock: Response of l-norepinephrine and isoproterenol. *J Clin Invest* 1977;49:1885–1902

7. Schleien CL, Dean JM, Koehler RC, Michael JR, Chantarojanasiri T, Traystman R, Rogers MC: Effect of epinephrine on cerebral and myocardial perfusion in an infant animal preparation of cardiopulmonary resuscitation. *Circulation* 1986;73:809–817

8. Brown CG, Werman HA: Adrenergic agonists during cardiopulmonary resuscitation. *Resuscitation* 1990;19:1–16

9. Zaritsky A, Nadkarni V, Getson P, Kuehl K: CPR in children. *Ann Emerg Med* 1987;16:1107–1111

10. Perkin RM, Levin DL, Webb R, Aquino A, Reedy J: Dobutamine: A hemodynamic evaluation in children with shock. *J Pediatr* 1982;100:977–983

11. Zaritsky AL, Chernow B: Catecholamines and other inotropes, in Chernow B (ed): *The Pharmacologic Approach to the Critically Ill Patient.* Baltimore, Williams & Wilkins, 1988, p 584

12. Zimmerman JJ, Dietrich KA: Current perspectives on septic shock. *Pediatr Clin North Am* 1987;34:131–163

13. Parker MM, Shelhamer JH, Bacharach SL, Green MV, Natanson C, Frederick TM, Damske BA, Parrillo JE: Profound but reversible myocardial depression in patients with septic shock. *Ann Intern Med* 1984;100:483–490

14. Chernow B, Roth BL: Pharmacologic manipulation of the peripheral vasculature in shock: Clinical and experimental approaches. *Circ Shock* 1986;18:141–155

15. Desjars P, Pinaud M, Bugnon D, Tasseau F: Norepinephrine therapy has no deleterious renal effects in human septic shock. *Crit Care Med* 1989;17:426–429

16. Desjars P, Pinaud M, Potel G, Tasseau F, Touze MD: A reappraisal of norepinephrine therapy in human septic shock. *Crit Care Med* 1987;15:134–137

17. Cunnion RE, Parrillo JE: Myocardial dysfunction in sepsis. *Crit Care Clin* 1989;5:99–118